Cookbook
of
Healthy
Living
&
No Regrets

Volume I, 2021
by Jayne J. Jones

Grab your oven mitts, aprons & join the No Sugar Baker team!

ISBN: 978-0-578-85769-5

Library of Congress Control Number: 2021902748

Printed in the United States of America

March 2021

Cover and Interior Design by Zalikha Zamri
Photography by SRQ Headshots

Published by The No Sugar Baker, LLC, Florida.

www.nosugarbaker.com

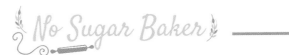
"To everyone on the No Sugar Baker Team, we are in this lifelong battle to good health together! I'm forever grateful, blessed and awed in joy to God for showing me the light, gifting me to be the light to others, and saving my life, and others."

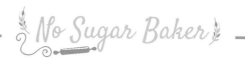

Table of Contents

Baking Station 1:

The Bitter Diagnosis, Leads to Savoury Lifestyle & Health

Baking Station 2:

Recipes for Healthy Living

No Sugar Baker's Brunch

No Sugar Baker's Bars, Cookies & Desserts

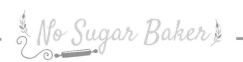

No Sugar Baker's Salads, Sides & Soups

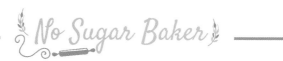

No Sugar Baker's Tasty Family Dinner Time Treats

No Sugar Baker's Party Zone

Baking Station 3:
Meet the No Sugar Baker Team

Baking Station 1:

The Bitter Diagnosis, Leads to Savoury Lifestyle & Health

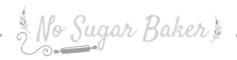
Baking Station 1:
Life is Sweet, No Bun Intended!

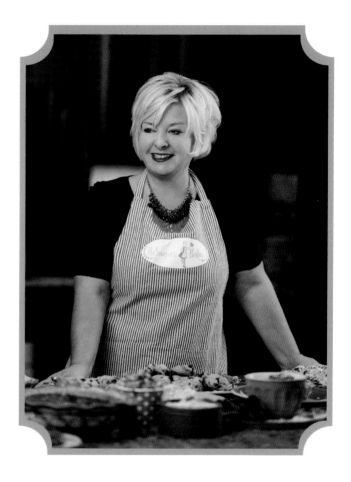

Sizzling toasty greetings! Welcome to my kitchen! I'm thrilled you are here and now are a part of the No Sugar Baker team! I promise you I will always be authentic and real. On my 45th birthday, I got oozing sick. I mean sick!

I found myself scraping the cream cheese frosting off a store-bought carrot cake. It was just me, the knife and the cake. I puked afterward and couldn't stay awake for the life of me. I told myself tomorrow was a new day. But, kept my poor habits.

Fast forward, two weeks later and nothing changed, except more puking, and me shoving in popsicles as fast as I could. The Hubs had enough. With a feisty wife, he didn't give in and dragged me to the Emergency Room. "We" got an eye-opening diagnosis, followed by a dreaded visit with my family physician. It was time. I rolled up my sleeves, put on my tennis shoes and put away my apron. I was determined to get my life back.

That was just over 18 months ago. Currently, I am diabetic prescription free. My A1C has dropped 7 points, my dress size has dropped 4 sizes. I've lost over 60 pounds. All by diet and exercise.

I'm back in my beloved kitchen baking sugar free and not missing a beat. I prefer to use Swerve. You can use whatever sweetener you prefer.

Grab your oven mitt and come along with me.

We're on a roll. Life is sweet. All this made with LOVE!

Jayne

(aka The No Sugar Baker!)

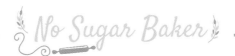
The Health Journey

This is hard to write. It's the hard-core truth. Time to face the oven, the heat is on.

About two years ago, I went cold turkey. I was determined that my constant stomach pain was from my habit of daily drinking 8-10 cans of diet soda. The stomach pains continued. Next up on the chopping block, I was determined that red meat was now making me sick. So, I went cold turkey again. The stomach pains continued.

Back to my 45th birthday and celebration. I had no energy to celebrate, but The Hubs being a genuine nice guy, insisted that we celebrate over an ice cream cone. We did. And, I got sick. From that night on, I struggled to eat without massive diarrhea. I'm not talking about a newborn's diaper of poo. I'm talking gut wrenching, tear flowing diarrhea. Over half of the time, I would run to the bathroom hoping to make it in time— unzipping my pants as I waddled to the toilet. Then, to roll back into bed.

I was looking forward to a summer trip we had planned with The Folks. But, I didn't want The Folks or The Hubs to know how miserable I actually was. The Hubs and I packed our bags. I think he secretly was praying I wouldn't have an accident on the airplane. On our layover, The Hubs asked if I was hungry. I replied, "Has that ever been a question?" He laughed. We found an airport greasy spoon diner.

After browsing the menu, I told him I wanted to order chicken fingers, fries and an Oreo shake. "Really? It's not even 9 am!" he asked. "Yes I'm craving a shake. You would, too, if you've thrown up for the past two weeks." I replied. He ordered the same. Yes, every patron around us looked on with envy and intrigue. Ok, more heavy on the intrigue—no pun intended.

We landed—whew no accidents. I made it! The Folks greeted us with plastic goodie bags

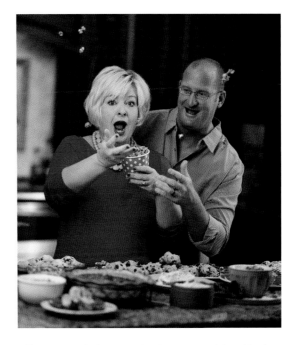

of homemade bars and other treats. It's a kind gesture and one very Minnesotan. At lunch, I told The Folks I've been sick with the "flu." But, I was on the mend and feeling better. The Folks said, "You are worn out and need to pace yourself. You work too hard." I didn't have the heart to tell them, I just spent two weeks in bed and was unable to function like an adult—let alone work. We carried on with our planned vacation. Yes, a vacation to a cooking and golf resort. What a coincidence. However, I didn't make it very long.

Almost daily, I found myself feeling okay in the morning and then early afternoon (post lunch) going from massive diarrhea to endless vomiting. Unlike me, I skipped every tour, cooking lesson and even a concert. Clearly, The Hubs and The Folks knew I had the "flu" and was downright sick. After The Hubs got back from a concert, I asked him to get me some regular cola soda. He looked puzzled but didn't question my yearlong pledge of no soda. He brought me three bottles. I downed them rapidly. I wanted three more bottles. He brought more.

The next day, The Folks flew home. We went

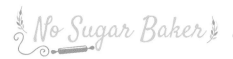

to Urgent Care. There, the nurse practitioner seemed stunned but finally opined I had a stomach infection. She prescribed an antibiotic. We went back to the resort. I didn't feel well. The Hubs brought me more regular soda. We had to fly home the next morning. I told The Hubs, I couldn't.

He politely said, "You have no choice. We need to get you home." I refused to eat or drink anything– as I was afraid of an accident on the airplane. As we waited in the airport security line, The Hubs held my shoulder as my body was trembling and physically shaking. My teeth were chattering. I couldn't even hold my hand still for the TSA agent. We flew and had a layover. I gasped seeing how many gates I needed to walk. We found a personal attendant with a wheelchair.

For the next week, the "flu" was vivid and getting worse. I had a craving. Popsicles. All I wanted to do was lick popsicles. Boxes of popsicles. Then, I'd find myself hurled over the toilet. Then, I'd eat another box of popsicles. The Hubs asked if he could go golfing. I felt selfish and guilty as he was my nurse for the past three weeks and he didn't leave the house. Surely, a grown independent woman could make it alone for a few hours?

When The Hubs returned, he found me endlessly vomiting in the kitchen sink. He asked how long I've been throwing up. I replied, "About four hours."

"That's it. We're going to the ER!" he ordered.

We arrived at the hospital. As we approached the emergency room entrance, I told The Hubs, "I'm fine. Let's go home." The Hubs said, "Not a f—ing chance. Get your ass in there."

And with that, our new life adventure began. Together, we walked into the emergency room.

The admitting nurse took my vital signs. "Are you on high blood pressure medicine?" "No, but it's always high. I feel fine." I replied. "Why aren't you? You cannot afford it? You can get it for free." she bluntly assumed.

"My blood pressure is always high," I said staring in disbelief at The Hubs. He lowered his hands motioning me to not rip into her comment. "You aren't going anywhere tonight. You are extremely sick," she informed me while printing my admitting bracelet. The Hubs and I looked at each other. We both surely were wondering what my concerning vital signs were. We got placed into an ER bed/ room. To save you agony and me some personal tears, I won't go into the nitty gritty details. We did find out, from nurse #3, my blood pressure on arrival was 285/175. My oxygen level was almost non-existent. I had a slight fever. For five hours, a rotating team of physicians, nurses and aides ran every test and screening imaginable.

The Hubs called The Folks right away. I think he wanted to talk to a reasonably sound mind, as we navigated this game of eliminating possible causes and illnesses. After the five hours, the head emergency room physician and lead RN came back into my room. They looked like they were about to deliver horrible news. "I have reached my evaluation. It's not good. You are severely diabetic." I looked at The Hubs—who shrugged his shoulders.

The physician continued, "Any of your grandparents or parents have diabetes?" I shrugged my shoulders and looked at The Hubs. He took that nonchalant clue and called The Folks instantly. "Well, it turns out, your paternal great-grandfather was diabetic, and your maternal grandmother had geriatric diabetes," he told all of us.

"Figures, diabetes skips a generation. You got a double whammy." she replied, "Your urine is full of spilled over sugar. Your glucose shows a sugar level

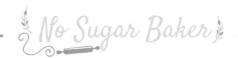

off the charts—over 12. You should be thankful you got here when you did." She left my bedside seemingly upset. The head nurse stayed behind and said, while squeezing my hand, "Kid, you are going to be okay. You are young. You have a wonderful husband and what it sounds like great parents. Get yourself a good doctor and follow their directions. It will be ok." She again squeezed my toe before leaving my bedside.

The ER physician returned. "I'm going to let you go home tonight. My final diagnosis is diabetes. You came to the ER saying you had a stomach infection—nothing related to diabetes. Therefore, I can't prescribe you any medication. You need to find a primary care doctor from this list. For now, eat salads and lean meats. Good luck to you."

We left, both feeling a sense of relief and ease. It was just diabetes and sounded like no problem. I had visions of still traveling that weekend to watch Em's first volleyball games of the season. Pretty easy—all I had to do was eat salads and lean meat. I was on it.

For forty-eight hours, The Hubs served up salads and lean meat only. I slept like a newborn. My body would shake, tremble and I felt like a drug addict detoxing. We supplemented meals with healthy snacks of grapes, apples and peanut butter, bananas, and salty crackers. Good sound choices, right?

I continued to vomit, shake and run to the bathroom. The next morning. "Damnit. Now I need a new phone," I told The Hubs, throwing my cell phone at him. He flicked on the tv for our usual weekend morning shows. "Can you see the tv?" I asked. He played with my phone and looked at me weird. "Nothing wrong with your phone. The tv is fine. What's wrong with you?" I rubbed my eyes.

"Everything is blurry." Within a few hours, my eyesight went from blurry to almost a zero ability to read, see or walk straight. I called a client of mine—an emergency room physician. After a full day of going back and forth between long telephone calls with him, he asked what my blood sugar was? "My blood sugar? I have no idea—how am I to know?" I asked. "You didn't get a meter from the ER? What medicine did they put you on? Tell The Hubs to go get you a blood glucose meter immediately. Check it in the morning and at night. Have him text me your numbers." That was midnight. The Hubs went shopping.

The next morning, like two anxious wannabe parents, we took my blood and stared at the device's screen waiting for the results. The prior evening, before bed, it was around 220. My friend/ the physician said it needed to be under 150 as he wasn't convinced, I was diabetic. It came back around 180 in the morning. "F—-" The Hubs remarked.

Both of us looked defeated. My friend/physician made an emergency prescription order of Metformin, to get me through until my first primary care appointment in 72 hours. I know that diabetes can affect anyone, from any walk of life. Currently, more than 30 million Americans have been diagnosed and 422 million people worldwide.

I'm not looking for sympathy or for you to cry me a river. Quite the contrary. I shared the diagnosis with a couple of friends and their reaction was… .."Oh diabetes—that's nothing—you'll be able to eat whatever you want. It's not a big deal. Get over it." I shouldn't have taken those words to heart. Well, this diagnosis isn't a life sentence of misery. It's been a wake-up call, a restart and a promise to myself for a happier and healthier life.

My first appointment with Doc Lopez I was scared shitless. I worried if my vision was ever coming

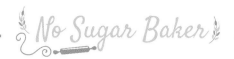

back. For the first time in my life, the clinic's scale wasn't the top stressor. It was the second stressor. The Hubs brought me into the clinic. He waited in the parking lot. The Folks waited by their phone.

Doc Lopez' Summary and Orders: 1. "You are lucky you didn't have a stroke. Your numbers are off the charts. You have an extremely high sugar count in your urine—that only happens when you've maxed out the blood range. You've been diabetic for years." 2. "We need to get you into an eye appointment immediately. Luckily, it seems like no other nerve or organ damage has happened. You got here and to the ER in the nick of time. Do you realize that?" 3. "If you listen, I can save your life. If not, you will die by the time you are fifty." 4. He drew a big circle onto the white paper of the patient bed. "Tell me what your dinner plate will look like?" I didn't understand. "Your plate, what's on that plate?" he asked. I shrugged my shoulders. "One half of every plate is going to be a lettuce salad with olive oil and lemon dressing, no other dressings. Ranch only in a tablespoon. Then ¼ of your plate is your protein—eat whatever meat you want at every meal. The other ¼ of the plate, a good carb only—like an exceedingly small potato or spoon of rice." 5. "I need you to drink half your body weight in water (ounces) every day. Nothing else and don't believe those diet teas—they are full of artificial flavoring— which means sugar. Anything that is flavored as orange, grape, peach are full of sugar. Even when it says its sugar free. Water." 6. "You need a 12 hour fast every 24-hour period. Don't eat anything after 7 pm and test your blood at night and in the morning. Keep track of your numbers—we need it at 100."

I questioned this and said my friend/physician said 150. "Are you going to listen to me or fight me?" he asked. 7. "You can't have more than 20 to 40 carbs a day. Your body can't process the sugar. That means absolutely no flour, sugar,

root vegetables—nothing from the ground, carrots, bananas, corn, peas, fruit, artificial sugars, peppers, milk, ice cream, yogurt, margarine, vegetable oil, bread and read all labels. Use regular butter, sour cream, salad, meat, eggs and cheese. Write out exactly what you eat and eat at least three times a day. Exercise. You must do something for only 20 minutes, 5 times a week." 8. "You are a mess—very unhealthy person. You will be seeing me every 20 days for now. Do you agree?"

He left the room. The nurse came in and said, "How'd it go?" "Not too bad—but I am still freaking out about my vision!" I got into our car. The Hubs knew not to ask many questions. I called The Folks—who listened, they didn't say anything, and ended the one-sided conversation with their standard, "Wonderful— just wonderful. Ok, um huh, wonderful." What no one knew is that I felt a tremendous amount of guilt, I was angry at myself for letting myself get to that point.

We got into a new routine—The Hubs would make breakfast and I would sulk. I would physically sit crying my eyes out for the first week—feeling so much guilt and hate towards myself. "I can't see you like this anymore—it's not you." he told me, asking how many eggs I wanted. We struggled together.

About my vision! I got a referral to an eye doctor from Doc Lopez. After attending that appointment, they gave me another referral to a retina specialist. The Hubs and I were shocked by their customer service, they told me to come in later that day. We went home to patiently wait. Patience has never been my strong suit, but The Hubs is the most relaxed person I know. Not that afternoon, he literally was pacing our kitchen and living room back and forth. We left for the appointment early, an hour early in fact.

I was nervous and still wasn't sure what was

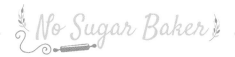

wrong with my eyesight. No one told me besides the urgency of going to the retina specialist. The Hubs escorted me into the eye clinic and told me, "No matter what, it will be okay." After a few routine eye scans and procedures, I was introduced to "Hot Doctor." A young trendy physician with genuine care and in comparison, a night and day difference in personality from Doc Lopez.

He too, though, didn't beat around the bush. Hot Doctor informed me I was "lucky" to get in when I did, or I'd be a girl with two detached retinas trying to salvage any eyesight left. He opined I needed a shot in each eye, once a month for the next twelve months. He also started in saying he was going to need to get my insurance approval before we did anything. I interrupted him, knowing the red tape of insurance bureaucracy, and said, "Don't worry about it. Let's do the shots now. I'll battle the insurance company later. " He replied, "I can't let you do that, Jayne. It's $4000 an eye, you need both eyes done for the next year or possibly more." I remember sitting in the patient chair, adding up the costs and risks. I was determined to tell him again, "We'll do it and worry about it later." Instead, Hot Doctor said, "I can get your insurance covered, give me a day."

I felt an enormous weight on my shoulders. I was scared for really one of the first times in my life. The Hubs came inside and helped me out to the car. When inside and alone, I told him the diagnosis. We both agreed that if we didn't hear from the insurance company within a day or two, we had no choice and needed to pay out of pocket. Within two hours of arriving home, Hot Doctor's office called saying they got the insurance approval. It was a Friday evening. I remember thinking I need to get through to Monday----hold on eyes—we can do it.

Instead, Hot Doctor had a different plan. We met at 8 am Saturday morning and the next morning as insurance regulations don't allow you to do both eyes on the same "date". Hot doctor told me,

"I'll see you in '30' days. Listen to Dr. Lopez. If anything goes wrong before then, you don't call me, you just show up."

30 days later. I shocked Hot Doctor. My eye scans and vision tests were almost normal, and he opined not to do another round of shots, as "we didn't want to waste any insurance approval if we didn't need to."

And, finally, we've reached the good part! I'm diabetic medicine free, 60 pounds lighter and have returned back to my kitchen, a place I came to despise for six months. I hesitated. I decided one day to make a no sugar cheeseburger soup. I brought a container of it to The Folks. They cried when they saw what I did and made. "What?" I asked, wondering what on earth got into them? "We've been waiting for this day. We've been praying for this day. Just wonderful. Absolutely wonderful."

I still have frequent "accidents" and if by mistake, I eat sugar even disguised as flour, oil, etc.—I get very sick.

Baking Station 2:

Recipes for Healthy Living

1. No Sugar Baker's Brunch

2. No Sugar Baker's Bars, Cookies & Desserts

3. No Sugar Baker's Salads, Sides & Soups

4. No Sugar Baker's Tasty Family
   Dinner Time Treats

5. No Sugar Baker's Party Zone

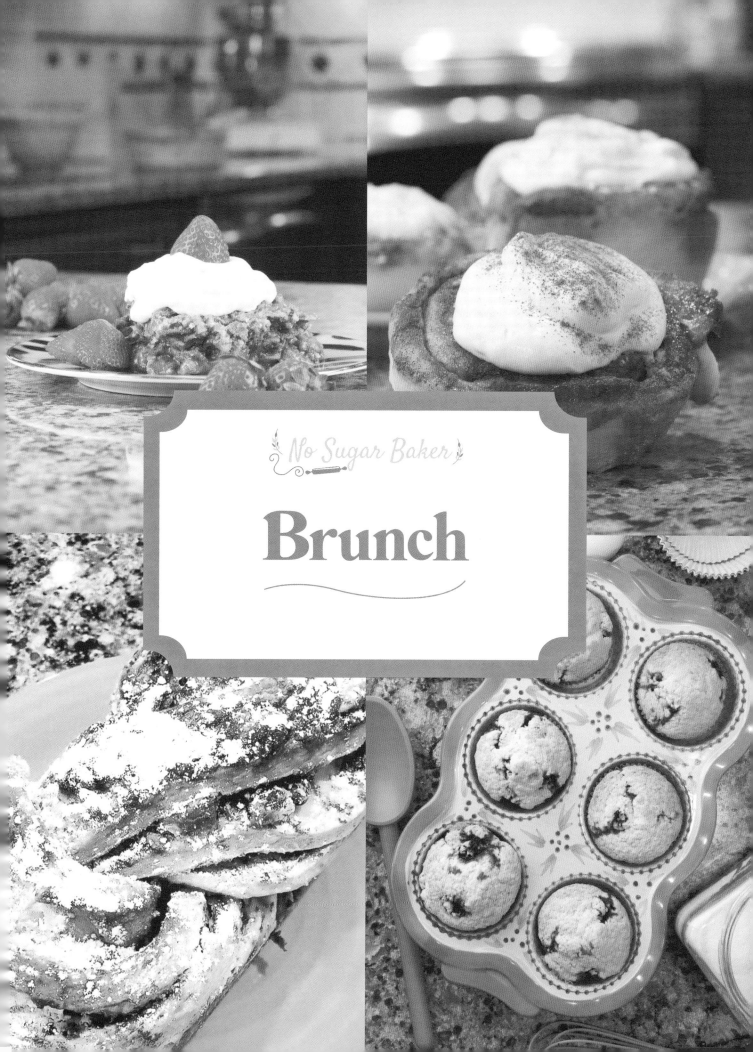

No Sugar Baker

Brunch

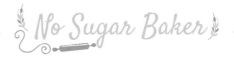

No Sugar Baker's Babka

Dough Ingredients:

¾ C. Unsweetened Almond Milk (Warmed to 90 degrees)

4 T. Butter

3 T. Swerve Granular

2 Egg Yolks + 2 Whole Eggs

1 T. Vanilla

4 C. Flour or Almond Flour

2 ½ t. Active Dry Yeast

Filling Ingredients:

1 C. Swerve Brown

2 T. Cinnamon

3 T. Melted Butter

Chopped Pecans to Sprinkle (Optional)

Easy Directions:

1. In bread machine, put dough ingredients in order in bread machine pan. Put on dough cycle.

2. When finished, place dough on floured surface and roll out into an 18x15 inch rectangle. Spread filling ingredients over dough.

3. Roll the dough, tightly—starting from one end of the long sides. Cut the roll in half, lengthwise, making two strands. Now, braid or twist the dough strands together. Try to keep the cut side on top, as much as possible.

4. You can shape your dough furthermore into a figure 8 shape. Place in a prepared greased and parchment lined 9x5 loaf pan. Let rise with warm towel on top of pan/dough for 30 minutes.

5. Bake at 350 for 30 minutes.

6. Let cool in pan for 10 minutes before removing. Serve with butter.

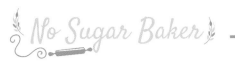

No Sugar Baker's Banana Cupcakes with Peanut Butter Frosting

Cupcake Ingredients:

¼ C. Butter

4 Oz. Cream Cheese

¾ C. Swerve Granular

4 Eggs

1 Tiny Small Banana

¼ C. Unsweetened Almond Milk

1 T. Vanilla

1 T. Banana Extract

2 ½ C. Flour

1 T. Baking Powder

Frosting Ingredients:

½ C. Melted Deli Fresh Peanut Butter

½ C. Butter

8 Oz. Cream Cheese (Room Temperature)

2 C. Swerve Confectioners

½ C. Heavy Whipping Cream

Easy Directions:

1. Prepare a cupcake pan with paper liners. Set aside.

2. In a large mixing bowl, combine first eight ingredients of cake recipe above.

3. After combined and well mixed, add in flour and baking powder. Mix thoroughly.

4. Fill each cupcake liner ¾ full. Bake at 325 for 15-20 minutes.

5. When cooled, prepare frosting. Whip or mix on high all frosting ingredients.

6. Spread heavily on top of cupcakes! Sweet!

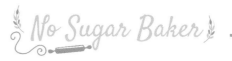
No Sugar Baker's Christmas Morning Blueberry Scones

Ingredients:
½ C. Frozen Butter
2 C. All Purpose or Almond Flour
½ C. Swerve Granular
2 ½ t. Baking Powder
1 t. Cinnamon

½ t. Salt
½ C. Heavy Whipping Cream
1 Egg
2 t. Vanilla
1 C. Fresh Blueberries

Easy Directions:

1. Grate frozen butter; then place in refrigerator while gathering the rest of the ingredients. For successful scones, you need COLD butter.

2. In a mixing bowl, whisk together flour, Swerve, baking powder, cinnamon and salt.

3. In another small bowl, mix cream, egg and vanilla.

4. Place all the ingredients from each above step in a food processor and pulse until the dough comes together.

5. Spoon the dough into another bowl, add in the blueberries. Place in refrigerator for at least 30 minutes to chill.

6. Line a cookie sheet with parchment paper. Lightly dust your countertop with flour. Remove dough from refrigerator. Pat the dough into a circular shape, about 8 to 10 inches in diameter. Then, cut the dough into 8 equal sized wedges. Using a spatula, place the wedges to your baking sheet. Top with extra cream lightly and sprinkle Swerve on top. Cover with plastic wrap and refrigerate overnight.

7. Bake at 400 for 20 minutes. Let cool. You can drizzle with a light icing made of Swerve Confectioners, cream cheese, cream and butter.

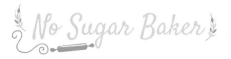

No Sugar Baker's
Chocolate Pumpkin Bread

Ingredients:

1 C. Flour or Almond Flour
½ C. Dark Cocoa
 2 t. Pumpkin Pie Spice
1 t. Baking Soda
½ t. Salt
1 15 Oz. Can Pumpkin Puree

1 C. Swerve Brown
½ C. Butter Melted
¼ C. Heavy Whipping Cream
2 Eggs
2 t. Vanilla
2 C. Lily's Dark Chocolate Chips

Easy Directions:

1. Spray a 9x5-inch loaf pan with non-stick cooking spray and set aside. In a medium bowl, whisk together the flour, cocoa powder, pumpkin pie spice, baking soda, and salt. Set aside.

2. In a large bowl, combine the pumpkin puree, Swerve Brown, melted butter, heavy cream, eggs, and vanilla extract.

3. Stir until smooth and combined. Stir the flour mixture in. Do not overmix. Add in 1 C. of the chocolate chips.

4. Pour batter into prepared pan. Sprinkle the remaining chocolate chips over the top of the bread.

5. Bake at 350 for 50-60 minutes. Let the bread cool in the pan for 15 minutes.

6. Run a knife around the edges of the bread. Remove the bread from the pan. Let the bread cool.

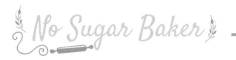

No Sugar Baker's
Banana Bread Without Bananas

Ingredients:

½ C. Butter

⅔ C. Swerve Granular

4 Eggs

1 T. Vanilla

1 T. Banana Extract

2 C. Almond or All Purpose Flour

5 t. Baking Powder

½ t. Xanthan Gum

2 t. Cinnamon

½ t. Salt

½ C. Sour Cream or Greek Yogurt

½ C. Chopped Walnuts or Pecans

½ C. Lily's Dark Chocolate Chips

Easy Directions:

1. Spray a 9x5 loaf pan and set aside.

2. In large bowl, cream together butter and Swerve.

3. Add in eggs, vanilla and banana extract.

4. In a separate small bowl, mix together flour, baking powder, xanthan gum, cinnamon and salt. When combined, add to the butter mixture.

5. Next, fold in the sour cream or Greek yogurt and combine well. Add in your walnuts, pecans and chocolate chips. Pour into pan.

6. Bake at 350 for 50-55 minutes. Remove from oven and let set in pan for 5-10 minutes.

7. Remove from pan and let cool. Slice and enjoy!

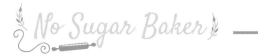

No Sugar Baker's Cinnamon Pecan Coffee Cake

Ingredients:

1 C. Butter

2 ¾ C. Swerve Granular, Divided

4 Eggs

2 C. Flour

1 T. Vanilla

1 t. Baking Soda

½ t. Salt

2 C. Sour Cream

2 T. Cinnamon

1 C. Chopped Pecans

Easy Directions:

1. In a large bowl, cream butter and 2 C. of Swerve until light and fluffy.

2. Add eggs, beating well after each one. Add in vanilla. Add in sour cream and mix until combined.

3. Mix together the flour, baking soda and salt. Pour slowly into batter and mix. In a small bowl, combine remaining Swerve, cinnamon and pecans.

4. Place a third of batter into a sprayed 10-in Bundt pan.

5. Sprinkle a third of Swerve/cinnamon/pecans mixture on top of batter. Repeat layering process two more times (three in total).

6. Bake at 350 for 45-50 minutes.

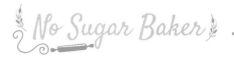
No Sugar Baker's
Hubs' Favorite Coffee Cake

Cinnamon Layer Ingredients:

¾ C. Swerve Brown

¾ C. Almond or All-Purpose Flour

1 T. Cinnamon

Crumb Topping Ingredients:

6 T. Butter, Melted

1 C. Swerve Brown

2 T. Cinnamon

1 C. Almond or All-Purpose Flour

Icing Ingredients:

1 C. Swerve Confectioners

4 T. Unsweetened Almond Milk

Cake Ingredients:

1 C. Butter

1 C. Swerve Granular

⅔ C. Swerve Brown

3 Eggs

2 T. Vanilla

¾ C. Sour Cream

½ t. Salt

3 t. Baking Powder

1 ¼ C. Unsweetened Almond Milk

3 ⅔ C. Almond or All-Purpose Flour

Easy Directions:

1. Spray a 9x13 baking dish and set aside. In a small bowl, whisk all the cinnamon layer ingredients and set aside.

2. In a second small bowl, mix all the crumb layer ingredients together. It will resemble crumbs and set aside. In a large mixing bowl, cream the butter, Swerve Granular and Swerve Brown, eggs, vanilla and sour cream.

3. Once mixed, add in the milk. Next add in the salt, baking powder and flour. Mix until combined.

4. Spread half of the cake batter into the prepared pan. Sprinkle the cinnamon layer filling over the batter. Next, carefully spread the remaining cake batter over the cinnamon layer. Sprinkle the crumb topping over the entire cake.

5. Bake at 350 for 40-45 minutes. Let slightly cool. You can make a glaze drizzle by mixing the icing ingredients in a small bowl and drizzle over the coffee cake. I sliced my pieces, placed on a serving plate and then, drizzled the glaze.

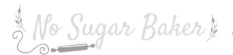

No Sugar Baker's
Pumpkin Caramel Rolls

Bread Machine Ingredients:
1 C. Unsweetened Almond Milk (Heat to 100 Degrees)
½ C. Water (About 110 Degrees—warm to the touch)
1 t. Cake Flavoring or Vanilla
½ C. Butter, Cut Into Pieces
2 Eggs (Room Temperature)
½ t. Salt
¾ C. Swerve Granular
5 C. Bread Flour (OR 3 C. Bread Flour and 2 C. Almond Flour)
3 t. Instant Active Yeast (I use Bread Machine Yeast)

Inner Roll Ingredients:
1 T. Cinnamon
4 Oz. Melted Cream Cheese
1 C. Pumpkin Puree
6 T. Melted Butter
1 T. Swerve Brown
1 T. Chopped Pecans

Cream Cheese Frosting Ingredients:
8 Oz. Cream Cheese (Room Temperature)
¾ C. Swerve Confectioners
1 T. Vanilla
2 T. Unsweetened Almond Milk

Easy Directions:

1. Put all bread machine ingredients in bread machine canister. Set on dough cycle.

2. When finished, remove dough from canister and put on lightly floured surface counter. Using rolling pin, roll out dough to ¼ inch thick.

3. In a small mixing bowl, combine melted cream cheese, pumpkin puree and melted butter. Spread onto dough. Heavily sprinkle with cinnamon and Swerve Brown.

4. Sprinkle chopped pecans. Starting from an outside edge, rollup dough tightly like a jelly roll. In a 9x12 baking pan, grease or spray baking pan and sprinkle with Swerve brown and additional cinnamon.

5. Cut dough into 12 even pieces. Place rolls into pan. Cover with a dish towel and let rise until double in size (about one hour).

6. Bake at 375 for 25-30 minutes. Let cool for 5 minutes and remove from pan. I made an easy cream cheese frosting by electric mixer using all the cream cheese frosting ingredients—spread onto cooled rolls.

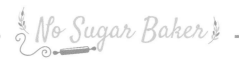

No Sugar Baker's
Triple Berry Scones

Ingredients:
2 C. Almond, Protein or All-Purpose Flour
½ C. Swerve Granular
1 T. Baking Powder
½ C. Butter (COLD)
1 Egg
½ C. Sour Cream
1 t. Vanilla

1 ½ C. Frozen or Fresh Mix of Berries (Strawberries, Blueberries, Raspberries or Blackberries)
¼ C. Swerve Confectioners

Easy Directions:

1. Line a baking sheet with parchment paper and set aside.

2. In a large mixing bowl, add flour, Swerve, baking powder. Combine.

3. Add in the butter and cut into pieces. You can easily use a food processor to make this dough.

4. Once butter is cut in, add egg, sour cream and vanilla. Continue to mix.

5. When combined, fold in berries. Roll out dough onto floured surface into a circle shape and cut into triangles.

6. Place on baking sheet. Bake at 400 for 15 minutes.

7. Let cool and top by sprinkling Swerve Confectioners!

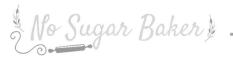
No Sugar Baker's
Blueberry Muffins

Topping Ingredients:
½ C. Almond Flour
½ C. Swerve Granular
½ t. Salt
4 T. Melted Butter

Filling Ingredients:
4 Oz. Cream Cheese
3 T. Swerve Granular

Batter Ingredients:
2 Eggs
1 C. Swerve Granular
8 T. Melted Butter
1 T. Vanilla
1 ½ t. Baking Soda
½ t. Salt
1 C. Sour Cream
2 C. Almond Flour or Bread Flour
1 Pint Fresh Blueberries

Easy Directions:

1. In a small bowl, combine all topping ingredients and set aside. In a large mixing bowl, mix eggs, Swerve, butter and vanilla.

2. Add in baking soda, salt and sour cream and mix till just blended. Add in flour. Combine gently and fold in blueberries.

3. In a separate mixing bowl, beat together cream cheese and Swerve.

4. Line a muffin baking pan with paper liners.

5. Using a spoon, fill each liner with batter measuring it half full. Then, add a small spoonful of the cream cheese mixture and finish by topping with a spoonful of batter.

6. Top each muffin with a spoonful of topping mixture. Bake at 350 for 20-25 minutes. Enjoy!

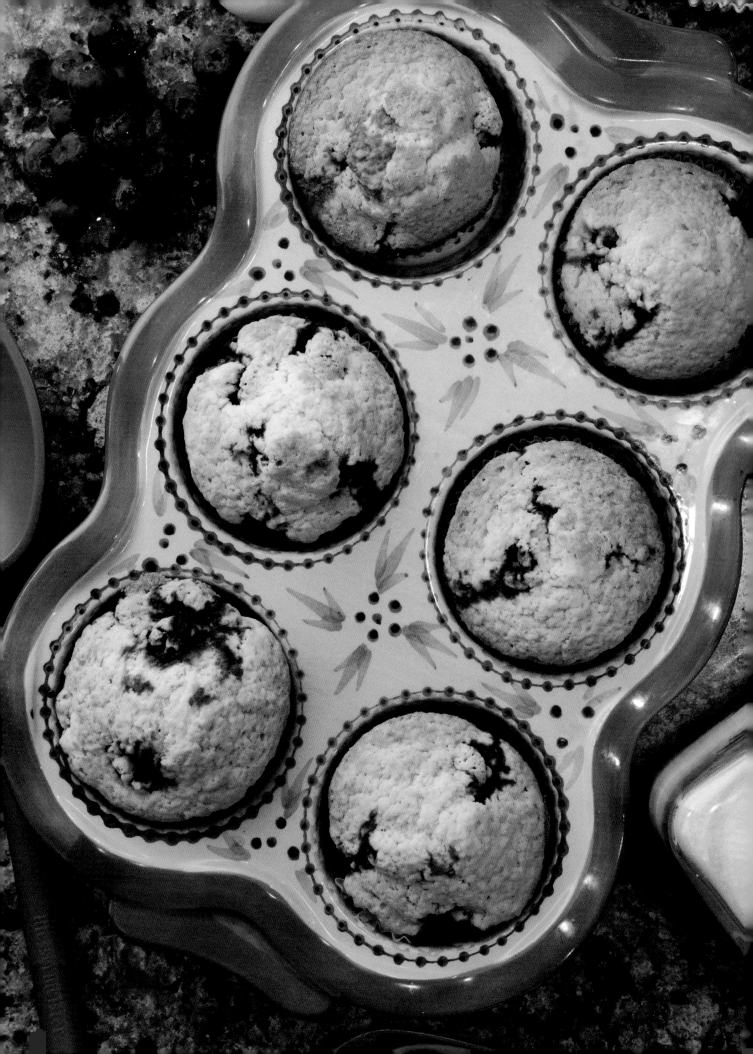

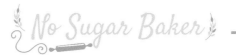

Brunch

No Sugar Baker's Waffles

Ingredients:

4 Eggs

4 Oz. Cream Cheese

½ C. Flour or Almond Flour

2 T. Melted Butter

1 T. Vanilla

1 T. Swerve Confectioners

1 t. Baking Powder

Easy Directions:

1. Mix all ingredients and pour into prepared waffle iron!

2. Top with your favorite no sugar syrup, strawberries and whipped cream! This is one of my new all-time favorites!

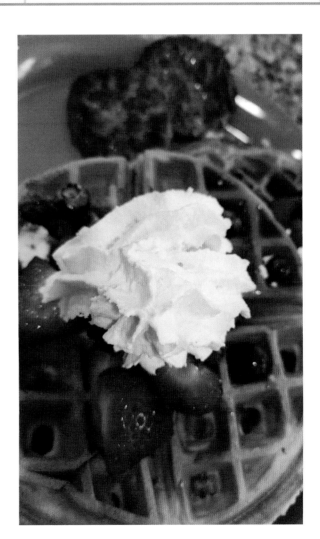

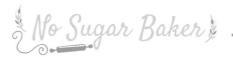

No Sugar Baker's
Strawberry Shortcake Slab

Filling Ingredients:
1 Pint Fresh Strawberries, Sliced
½ C. Swerve Granular
1 T. Lemon Juice

Whipped Cream Ingredients:
2 C. Heavy Whipping Cream
1 T. Vanilla
½ C. Swerve Confectioners

Cake Ingredients:
3 ½ C. Flour or Almond Flour
½ C. Swerve Granular
5 t. Baking Powder
½ t. Salt
1 C. Cold Butter, Cut Into Pieces
2 Eggs
2 C. Heavy Whipping Cream

Easy Directions:

1. Spray and line a 15x10 inch baking pan. In large bowl, mix together flour, Swerve, salt, and baking powder.

2. With two knives, cut in butter pieces, making crumbles. Mix in eggs and whipping cream. Pour into prepared pan. Bake at 400 for 16-18 minutes. Let cool.

3. While cooling, in a small bowl, combine all strawberries ingredients, stir and store in refrigerator.

4. When ready to serve, in a mixing bowl, whip together all whipped cream ingredients.

5. Put whipped cream onto cake, then add strawberry mixture. Pretty! Enjoy!

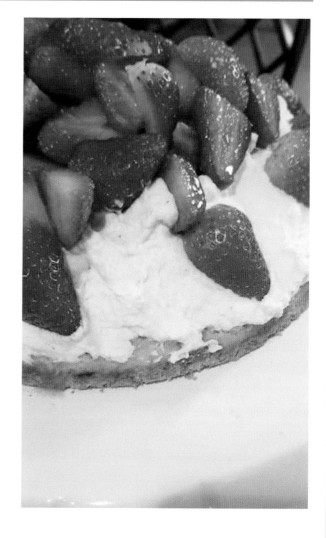

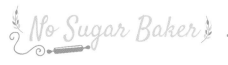

No Sugar Baker's
Cinnamon Rolls

Bread Machine Ingredients:
1 C. Unsweetened Almond Milk (Heat to 110 Degrees)
½ C. Water (About 110 Degrees—warm to the touch)
1 t. Cake Flavoring or Vanilla
½ C. Butter, Cut Into Pieces
2 Eggs (Room Temperature)
½ t. Salt
¾ C. Swerve Granular
5 C. Bread Flour (OR 3 C. Bread Flour and 2 C. Almond Flour)
3 t. Instant Active Yeast (I use Bread Machine Yeast)

Inner Roll Ingredients:
1 T. Cinnamon
4 Oz. Melted Cream Cheese
6 T. Melted Butter
1 T. Swerve Brown
1 T. Chopped Pecans

Cream Cheese Frosting Ingredients:
8 Oz. Cream Cheese (Room Temperature)
¾ C. Swerve Confectioners
1 T. Vanilla
2 T. Unsweetened Almond Milk

Easy Directions:

1. Put all bread machine ingredients in bread machine canister. Set on dough cycle.

2. When finished, remove dough from canister and put on lightly floured surface counter. Using rolling pin, roll out dough to ¼ inch thick.

3. In a small mixing bowl, combine melted cream cheese and melted butter. Spread onto dough. Heavily sprinkle with cinnamon and Swerve Brown. Sprinkle chopped pecans.

4. Starting from an outside edge, rollup dough tightly like a jelly roll. In a 9x12 baking pan, grease or spray baking pan and sprinkle additional cinnamon. Cut dough into 12 even pieces.

5. Place rolls into pan. Cover with a dish towel and let rise until double in size (about one hour). Bake at 375 for 25-30 minutes.

6. Let cool for 5 minutes and remove from pan. I made an easy cream cheese frosting by electric mixer using all the cream cheese frosting ingredients—spread onto cooled rolls.

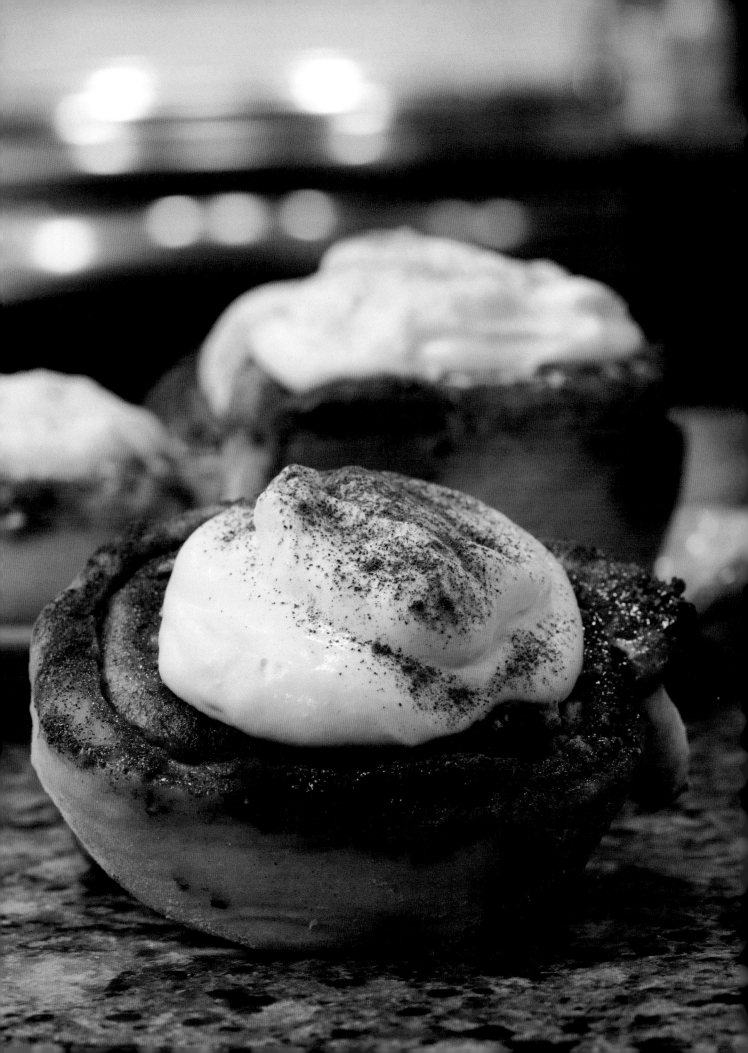

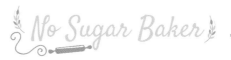

No Sugar Baker's
Blueberry Cream Cheese Coffeecake

Ingredients:

½ C. Butter

1 Egg

1 C. Heavy Whipping Cream

1 ½ C. Flour or Almond Flour

3 t. Baking Powder

½ t. Salt

1 C. Swerve Granular

4 C. Fresh Blueberries

8 Oz. Cream Cheese

Easy Directions:

1. In 8x10 baking dish, place butter.

2. Put into oven at 350 and melt butter. In a mixing bowl, combine all ingredients but blueberries and cream cheese.

3. After butter is melted, spread butter throughout pan. Pour batter onto butter.

4. Pat blueberries onto batter.

5. Cut cream cheese into small chunks and place – making sure that every angle has cream cheese.

6. Bake for 45 minutes. Serve warm! Watch out—this is yummy!!

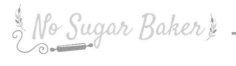

No Sugar Baker's
Strawberry Rhubarb Jam

Ingredients:
3 C. Diced Strawberries
2 C. Diced Rhubarb
1 C. Swerve Granular
2 T. Lemon Juice
2 T. Pectin

Easy Directions:

1. In a small bowl, combine all ingredients. Pour into bread machine canister.

2. Hit "Jam" cycle. When completed, remove from bread machine and pour into small sterilized jars.

3. Let cool. Seal with jar covers and store in refrigerator. The jam will keep for 5-7 days.

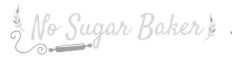

No Sugar Baker's
Cinnamon Chocolate Chip Bread

Ingredients:

2 T. Cinnamon
½ C. Swerve Granular
2 C. Almond Flour
2 t. Baking Soda
½ t. Salt
1 Egg
½ C. Swerve Brown

½ C. Swerve Granular
1 C. Heavy Whipping Cream
½ C. Melted Butter or ½ C. Vegetable Oil
1 T. Vanilla
2 C. Lily's Dark Chocolate Chips

Easy Directions:

1. In a small bowl, mix the Swerve Granular and cinnamon. Set aside.

2. In another small bowl, mix the flour, soda, salt and set aside.

3. In a large mixing bowl, combine the egg, Swerve Brown, Swerve Granular, cream, butter or oil and vanilla. Add in flour mixture.

4. When mixed slightly, fold in chocolate chips. In sprayed prepared (or well-greased) bread pan pour half of dough mixture.

5. Next sprinkle half of the cinnamon granular mixture onto dough.

6. Top with remaining dough and finish sprinkling remaining amount of cinnamon granular.

7. Bake at 350 for 60 minutes. Enjoy!

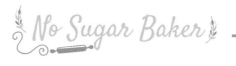

No Sugar Baker's
Chocolate Chip Muffins

Ingredients:

3 C. Flour or Almond Flour
4 t. Baking Powder
½ t. Baking Soda
½ t. Salt
2 t. Cinnamon
½ t. Nutmeg
¾ C. Melted Butter

1 C. Swerve Granular
2 Eggs
½ C. Sour Cream
1 C. Heavy Whipping Cream
1 T. Vanilla
2 C. Lily's Dark Chocolate Chips

Easy Directions:

1. In a small bowl, mix the flour, baking powder, baking soda, salt, cinnamon and nutmeg. Set aside.

2. In a large mixing bowl, mix butter, Swerve, eggs until well blended.

3. Add in sour cream, whipping cream and vanilla. Add in flour mixture and stir until slightly combined.

4. Toss in the chocolate chips. Spray or paper line a cupcake pan.

5. You can either make small sized muffins or large muffins. Fill pan and sprinkle a little extra Swerve and cinnamon on top of each muffin.

6. Bake at 425 for 5 minutes, then reduce heat to 350 for another 25 minutes.
   .

7. Let cool for a few minutes and enjoy!

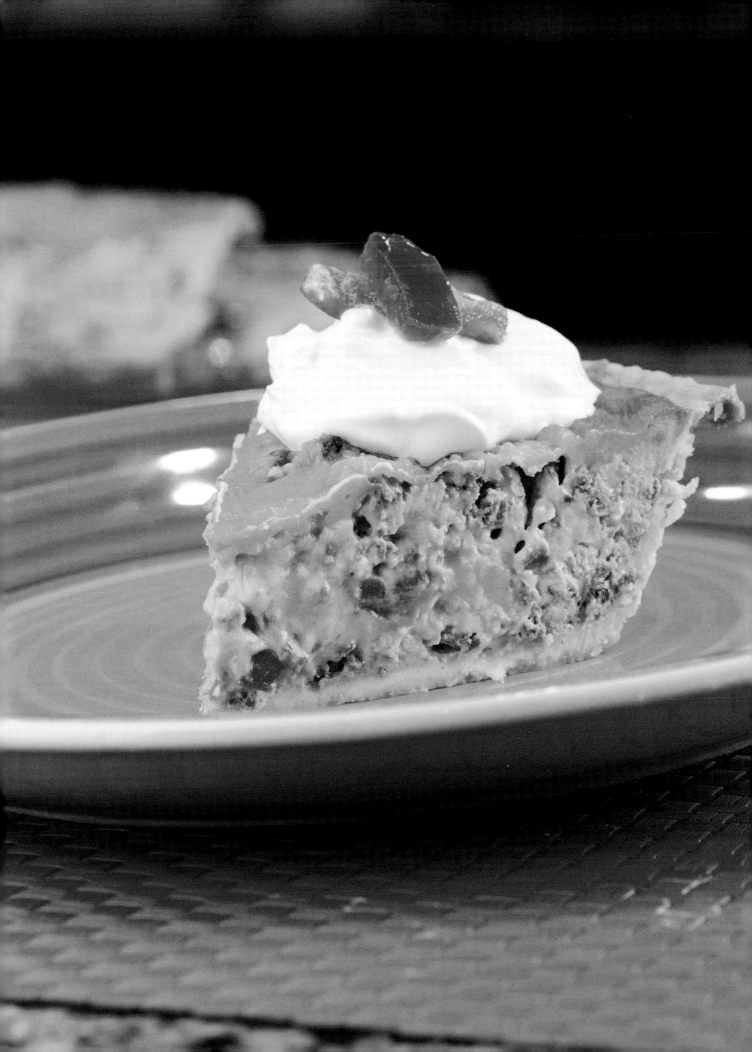

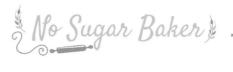
The No Sugar Baker's
Cheeseburger Quiche

Ingredients:

1 ½ Lbs. Ground Beef

4 Slices Bacon

½ C. Diced Onion

1 T. Garlic Powder

Salt and Pepper to Taste

1 T. Onion Powder

6 Eggs

¼ C. Mustard

½ C. Mayonnaise

½ C. Heavy Whipping Cream

2 C. Shredded Cheddar Cheese

½ C. Shredded Mozzarella Cheese

Easy Directions:

1. Cook the bacon and ground beef in large skillet, until no longer pink. Add in onion, salt and pepper, garlic powder and onion powder.

2. Cook for an additional five minutes, drain pan drippings and discard. Then, place mixture into greased pie pan.

3. Spread 1 C. cheddar cheese and all mozzarella cheese on top of meat. In a mixing bowl, mix eggs, mayonnaise, mustard and whipping cream.

4. When combined, pour on top of cheese. Next, top with remaining cheddar cheese.

5. Bake at 350 for 40 minutes.

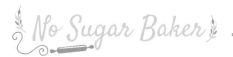
No Sugar Baker's Blueberry Cheesecake Coffeecake

Coffeecake Layer Ingredients:
1 ½ C. Almond Flour
1 t. Baking Powder
1 t. Baking Soda
½ t. Salt
6 T. Butter
½ C. Swerve Granular
1 Egg + 1 Egg Yolk
¾ C. Sour Cream
1 T. Vanilla
1 C. Fresh Blueberries

Cheesecake Layer Ingredients:
½ C. Swerve Granular
16 Oz. Cream Cheese
2 Egg Whites
1 T. Vanilla
2 C. Fresh Blueberries

Sugary Crunch Layer Ingredients:
½ C. Swerve Granular
½ C. Flour or Almond Flour
4 T. Cold Butter, Cut Into Cubes

Easy Directions for Coffeecake Layer:

1. In a small mixing bowl, combine flour, baking powder, baking soda and salt. Set aside. In a mixing bowl, mix butter, Swerve, eggs, and vanilla.

2. Add in one half of the flour mixture and stir. Add in one half of the sour cream and stir. Continue with the rest of the flour mixture and stir gently.

3. Continue with the remaining sour cream and stir gently. Pour into a well-greased, parchment paper lined 9-inch springform pan or round pan. Top mixture with fresh blueberries. Set aside.

Easy Directions for Cheesecake Layer:

1. In a mixing bowl, whip on high Swerve, cream cheese, egg white and vanilla. When smooth and combined, fold in blueberries. Pour onto the cake layer and, if you choose, place more blueberries on top. Set aside.

Easy Directions for Sugary Crunchy Layer:

1. Combine all ingredients in a small bowl, using a fork or your hands, make a crumbly mixture. Put onto cake. Bake at 350 for 45-55 minutes. Set in refrigerator to cool and let set for at least 3 hours.

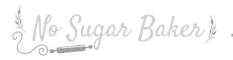

No Sugar Baker's Raspberry Cream Cheese Rolls

Dough Ingredients:
1 C. Butter
8 Oz. Cream Cheese
2 C. Almond Flour

Filling Ingredients:
1 C. Fresh Raspberries
¼ C. Swerve Granular
¼ C. Water

¼ C. Cornstarch
½ C. Sliced Almonds
4 Oz. Cream Cheese

Cream Cheese Frosting Ingredients:
8 Oz. Cream Cheese (Room Temperature)
½ t. Vanilla
½ C. Swerve Confectioners
1 T. Heavy Whipping Cream

Easy Directions:

1. In a mixing bowl, cream butter and cream cheese. Add in flour and mix. Dough will form and set into a ball. Wrap in plastic wrap and refrigerate for an hour.

2. While dough is chilling move onto the filling. Place raspberries, water and Swerve into a saucepan. Bring to boil and stir for 2-3 minutes.

3. Remove from heat, add in cornstarch. Stir until smooth, set aside and let cool. When cooled, stir in cream cheese and combine.

4. Roll out dough into rectangle with floured rolling pin. Spread the raspberry filling down the center of the dough, sprinkle sliced almonds on top.

5. You will want to leave a ½" border. Tightly roll the dough lengthwise. Cut the dough into 15-20 slices. Place slices cut-side down on baking sheet lined with parchment paper. Bake at 375 for 16 minutes, or until golden brown.

6. Let the rolls cool. You can add a cream cheese frosting to add some spark. Combine all ingredients and mix until the frosting is formed. For added presentation you can sprinkle a few almond slices!

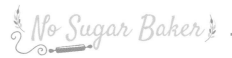

No Sugar Baker's
Pumpkin Pecan and Chocolate Bread

Ingredients:

2 ¼ C. Almond Flour
½ t. Salt
1 t. Cinnamon
½ t. Nutmeg
¾ C. Swerve Granular
1 ¼ t. Baking Soda
2 Beaten Eggs

½ C. Butter, Melted
1 ¼ C. Pumpkin Puree
¾ C. Chopped Pecans
½ C. Lily's Dark Chocolate Chips

Easy Directions:

1. Blend together: flour, salt, cinnamon, nutmeg, Swerve, and baking soda in a large mixing bowl. Add eggs, butter and pumpkin puree continuing to gently mix until smooth and combined.

2. Add pecans and chocolate chips. Pour into a standard sprayed/greased loaf pan.

3. Bake at 350 for 30 minutes or until toothpick comes out clean. Let cool. Serve and enjoy.

4. P.S. I did make a cream cheese frosting with Swerve Confectioners, cream cheese and a tad bit of heavy cream. It was a bit rich for this bread, butter on this treat is delicious!

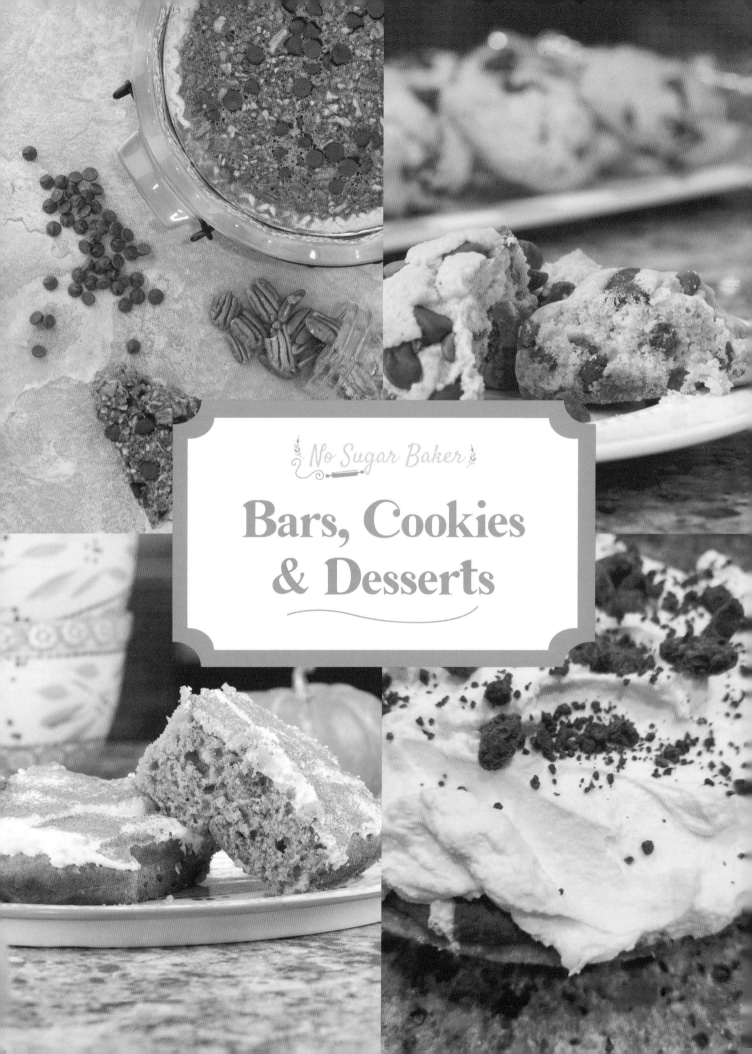

No Sugar Baker

Bars, Cookies & Desserts

No Sugar Baker's
Popcorn Cookies

Ingredients:

½ C. Butter

2 C. Swerve Granular

1 Egg

1 T. Vanilla

1 ¼ C. Flour or Almond Flour

½ t. Baking Soda

Dash of Salt

2 C. Popped Popcorn, Slightly Crushed

1 C. Lily's Dark Chocolate Chips

½ C. Chopped Pecans

Easy Directions:

1. In a mixing bowl, cream butter, Swerve, egg and vanilla.

2. Add in flour, baking soda and salt. Mix.

3. Fold in popcorn, chocolate chips and pecans. Place on greased or parchment paper lined cookie sheet.

4. Bake at 350 for 10 minutes.

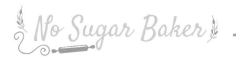

No Sugar Baker's Strawberry Angel Food Cookies

Ingredients:
1 Angel Food Cake Mix
¾ C. Sugar Free Strawberry Preserves
3 T. Mini Lily's Dark Chocolate Chips

Easy Directions:

1. In a mixing bowl, mix cake mix and preserves until moistened.

2. Add in chocolate chips. Line a cookie sheet with parchment paper and drop dough onto sheet.

3. You can sprinkle with sliced almonds. Bake at 325 for 11 minutes. Cookies will be soft and chewy!

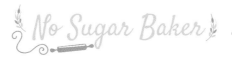

No Sugar Baker's
Vanilla Pudding

Ingredients:

⅓ C. Swerve Brown

2 ½ T. Cornstarch

2 C. Half & Half

2 Egg Yolks

2 T. Butter

1 t. Vanilla

Easy Directions:

1. In microwave safe bowl, combine Swerve and cornstarch. Add in half & half and egg yolks. Mix well.

2. Microwave for 5 minutes. Whisk well to prevent lumps.

3. Again, microwave for 2 additional minutes. Stir in butter and vanilla. If the pudding appears to have lumps, beat well.

4. Pour into dessert dishes and refrigerate. You can top your pudding with whipped cream, almonds, chocolate chips or berries.

5. Variation: You can substitute unsweetened almond milk for the half & half.

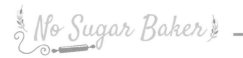

Bars, Cookies & Desserts

No Sugar Baker's Sweet Tooth Holiday Treat

Ingredients 1:	**Ingredients 2:**
¼ C. Butter	½ t. Pink Himalayan Salt or Salt
1 Pkg. Lily Semi-Sweet Chocolate Baking Chips Made With Stevia	2 C. Sliced Almonds
½ C. Swerve Brown	

Easy Directions:

1. In a small bowl, microwave all ingredients under "Ingredients #1" until melted and you can stir it.

2. Next, pour in all ingredients under "Ingredients #2" and combine.

3. Spoon the batter onto a parchment paper lined cookie sheet and refrigerate until firm.

No Sugar Baker's Brown Sugar Blondies

Blondies Ingredients:
½ C. Butter
2 C. Swerve Brown
2 Eggs
2 t. Vanilla
2 ⅔ C. All-Purpose or Almond Flour
2 t. Baking Powder
½ t. Salt

Blondies Frosting Ingredients:
½ C. Swerve Brown
½ C. Butter
4 Oz. Cream Cheese

Easy Directions:

1. Spray a 9x13 baking pan. In a mixing bowl, cream together butter, Swerve, eggs and vanilla.

2. Add in flour, baking powder and salt. Blend well. Bake at 350 for 35 minutes.

Easy Directions for Blondies Frosting:

1. Mix ingredients well. Spread on blondies and sprinkle with sugar free sprinkles!

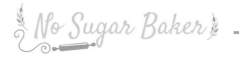

No Sugar Baker's
Spritz

Ingredients:

1 C. Butter

4 Oz. Cream Cheese

1 C. Swerve Granular

1 Egg Yolk

1 T. Vanilla

2 ½ C. Flour or Almond Flour

½ t. Salt

1 t. Cinnamon

Little Orange Zest

Green and Red Food Coloring

Easy Directions:

1. In a mixing bowl, cream butter, cream cheese and Swerve until light and fluffy. Add in egg yolk and vanilla.

2. Add in flour, salt and cinnamon, Stir in orange zest and food coloring of choice.

3. You can roll cookies or use a cookie press. Bake on cookie sheet lined with parchment paper.

4. Bake at 350 for 9-10 minutes.

No Sugar Baker's Angel Food Coconut Macaroons

Ingredients:
1 C. Cold Water
1 Angel Food Cake Mix
6 C. Unsweetened Shredded Coconut

Easy Directions:

1. In a clean, grease-free mixing bowl, pour water and add cake mix.

2. Whisk until well blended, then fold in the coconut.

3. Scoop batter into small balls by using a spoon or small ice cream scoop.

4. Place on parchment paper lined baking sheet. Bake at 350 for 20 minutes.

5. Do not overbake. Allow to cool.

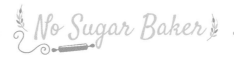

No Sugar Baker's
Jam Thumbprints

Ingredients:
1 C. Butter, Softened
⅔ C. Swerve Granular
2 Egg Yolks
1 t. Vanilla
¼ t. Salt
2 ⅓ C. Flour

1 Small Jar Unsweetened Jam

Easy Directions:

1. In a mixing bowl, combine butter, Swerve, egg yolks and vanilla. Fold in salt and flour.

2. Shape dough into balls.

3. Make an indentation in each cookie using your thumb. Then fill each indent with ½ t. of unsweetened jam.

4. Bake at 350 for 12-14 minutes. Do not over bake.

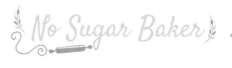

No Sugar Baker's
Sugar Cookies Made By Mom

Ingredients:
2 ¾ C. Flour
1 t. Baking Soda
½ t. Baking Powder
1 C. Butter
1 ½ C. Swerve Granular
1 Egg
1 t. Almond Flavoring

Icing Ingredients:
½ C. Butter
8 Oz. Cream Cheese (Room Temperature)
4 C. Swerve Confectioners
2 t. Vanilla or Almond Flavoring

Easy Directions:

1. In a mixing bowl, combine butter, Swerve, egg and almond flavoring. In a small bowl, combine flour, baking soda and baking powder. Add this mixture to batter.

2. Using a spoon or small scoop form the batter into small balls.

3. Place on a baking sheet. With a lightly floured fork, push each ball down slightly. Bake at 375 for 7-8 minutes or until golden brown. Remove and let cool.

4. Make a icing by whipping together all icing ingredients until light and fluffy.

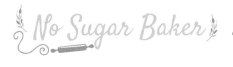

No Sugar Baker's
Chocolate Pin Wheels

Ingredients:
4 Oz. Cream Cheese
¼ C. Butter
½ C. Swerve Granular
1 1/8 C. Flour
¼ t. Baking Soda
1 t. Vanilla
½ C. Lily's Dark Chocolate Chips

Easy Directions:

1. In a mixing bowl, combine cream cheese, butter and Swerve. In a small bowl, combine flour and baking soda. Add this mixture to the batter and add in vanilla.

2. Divide dough into half. To one of the halves, add chocolate chips and mix well.

3. Chill the two halves in the refrigerator. Roll dough half out separately on a floured surface into a rectangular shape. Place the light-colored rectangle on top of the chocolate colored rectangle. At the narrow end roll into a jelly roll shape. Wrap the dough in plastic wrap and refrigerate overnight.

4. Slice the dough into ¼ inch slices and lay on cookie sheet. Bake at 350 for 10 minutes.

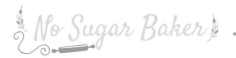
No Sugar Baker's
Cranberry Blueberry Pie

Ingredients:

1 Baked Pie Crust (Use No Sugar Baker's recipe!)

¼ C. Vodka

1 C. Water

1 C. Fresh Blueberries

2 ½ C. Fresh Cranberries

1 T. Unflavored Gelatin

1 t. Orange Zest

1 t. Ground Ginger

½ C. Swerve Granular

8 Oz. Cream Cheese

1 ½ C. Cold Heavy Cream

Top with No Sugar Baker's Whipped Cream Recipe

Easy Directions:

1. In a large saucepan, bring vodka, water, Swerve, blueberries and cranberries to boil. Let boil for 6 minutes.

2. Remove from heat and add in gelatin, orange zest and ginger. Stir until dissolved. Let cool.

3. In a large mixing bowl, beat cream cheese and heavy whipping cream.

4. Add in cranberry/blueberry mixture and fold until smooth. Pour into pie crust and refrigerate overnight.

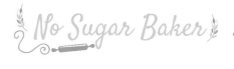
No Sugar Baker's
Pecan Pie Brownies

Ingredients:

4 Eggs
1 ¼ C. Cocoa
1 T. Vanilla
½ t. Salt
1 t. Baking Powder
1 C. Butter
2 ¼ C. Swerve Granular
1 ½ C. All-Purpose Flour or Almond Flour
1 C. Lily's Dark Chocolate Chips

¾ C. Swerve Brown
½ C. Sugar Free Breakfast Syrup
½ C. Melted Butter
1 T. Salt
2 Eggs
1 T. Bourbon
3 ½ C. Chopped Pecans

Easy Directions:

1. Spray a 9x9 inch baking pan and line with parchment paper. In a mixing bowl, combine the eggs, cocoa, vanilla, salt, and baking powder.

2. In a separate bowl, melt butter and add the Swerve, stir until dissolved. Add the butter mixture to the first bowl.

3. Mix and add in the flour and chocolate chips. Stir batter until smooth. Pour batter into pan and bake at 350 for 30-35 minutes.

4. In a small bowl, whisk together the Swerve Brown, syrup, melted butter, vanilla, salt, eggs and bourbon.

5. Add in the pecans. Stir. Gently pour the pecan mixture over the baked brownie.

6. Bake until the pecan layer is golden (about 30 minutes). Let cool completely overnight.

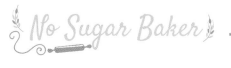
No Sugar Baker's
The Best Pumpkin Pie

Ingredients:

1 Unbaked Pie Crust

8 Oz. Cream Cheese

1 15 Oz. Can Pumpkin Puree

½ C. Melted Butter

3 Eggs

3 ¼ C. Swerve Confectioners

1 t. Cinnamon

1 t. Nutmeg

¼ t. Salt

Top with No Sugar Baker's Whipped Cream Recipe

Easy Directions:

1. In a mixing bowl, beat the cream cheese until light and fluffy. Add in the pumpkin and mix again.

2. Add in the melted butter and vanilla. Add eggs mixing well after each one.

3. Add Swerve Confectioners, and spices.

4. Bake at 400 for 15 minutes, reduce oven heat to 350 and bake for another 40-45 minutes. Let chill in refrigerator for at least 4 hours.

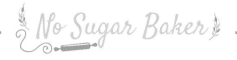

No Sugar Baker's
Easy Cranberry Crunch

Ingredients:

24 Oz. Fresh Cranberries

1 C. Swerve Brown

½ C. Lemon Juice

1 T. Vanilla

1 C. Chopped Pecans

1 C. Slivered Almonds

½ C. Swerve Brown

¼ C. All-Purpose or Almond Flour

⅓ C. Melted Butter

2 T. Cinnamon

Easy Directions:

1. Spray a 9x9 baking dish OR individual small baking ramekins and set aside. In saucepan, bring cranberries, 1 C. Swerve Brown, and lemon juice to a rolling boil.

2. Remove from heat and add in vanilla. Let sit for 5 minutes.

3. In a small bowl, combine pecans, almonds, remaining Swerve Brown, flour, cinnamon and melted butter until crumbly.

4. Place the cranberry mixture into the bottom of the baking pan or each ramekin. Top with crumbly topping. Bake at 350 for 30 minutes.

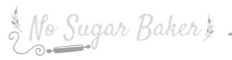

No Sugar Baker's
Turtle Cheesecake

Crust Ingredients:
1 C. All-Purpose or Almond Flour
⅓ C. Swerve Brown
¼ C. Chopped Pecans
6 T. Chilled Butter, Cubed

Cheesecake Ingredients:
32 Oz. Cream Cheese
1 C. Swerve Granular
⅓ C. Swerve Brown
¼ C. All-Purpose or Almond Flour (+ 1 t.)
3 T. Heavy Whipping Cream
1 T. Vanilla

4 Eggs
1 C. Lily's Dark Chocolate Chips, Melted
¼ Sugar Free Caramel Sauce OR (Make No Sugar Baker's Caramel Sauce by bringing to a boil 1 C. Swerve Brown, ½ C. Sugar Free Maple Breakfast Syrup and ½ C. No Sugar Caramel Coffee Syrup—remove from boiling heat and add in 1 T. Vanilla and 1 T. Cornstarch)
½ C. Chopped Pecans

Easy Directions:

1. Spray a 9-in springform pan. In a small bowl, combine all the crust ingredients until crumbly. Press into bottom of the pan. Bake at 325 for 15 minutes.

2. Set aside and let cool. In a large mixing bowl, beat cream cheese and both Swerves until creamy. Beat in ¼ C. flour, cream and vanilla.

3. Add eggs and mix well. Remove 1 cup of batter to a small bowl and stir in melted chocolate chips. Spread this chocolate layer over the crust. In another small bowl, mix your caramel sauce with 1 t. flour and pecans. Add this layer to the cheesecake. Top with remaining cheesecake batter.

4. Bake at 325 for 75-80 minutes. Cool for 10 minutes on kitchen countertop. Loosen sides from pan with a knife and let cool for another 60 minutes.

5. Place in refrigerator overnight. When ready to serve, you can add extra whipped cream, pecans and caramel sauce! Delightful!

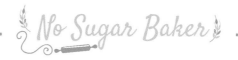

No Sugar Baker's
Chocolate Almond Butter Bread

Ingredients:

4 Eggs

1 C. All Natural Almond Butter

1 t. Baking Powder

3 T. Unsweetened Cocoa

4 T. Lily's Dark Chocolate Chips

4 T. Swerve Granular

2 t. Vanilla

Pinch of Salt

Easy Directions:

1. In large bowl, whisk the eggs and baking powder.

2. Next add in the almond butter, cocoa, Swerve, salt and vanilla, mixing until well combined.

3. Fold in the chocolate chips. Spoon into a well sprayed 9x5 loaf pan. Bake at 350 for 25 minutes!

No Sugar Baker's
Cinnamon Twirl Cookies

Ingredients:

1 C. Butter

1 C. Sour Cream

1 Egg Yolk

2 ½ C. All-Purpose Flour or Almond Flour

Salt (A Pinch)

1 C. Chopped Pecans or Walnuts

1 C. Swerve Granular

3 t. Cinnamon

1 T. Swerve Confectioners

Easy Directions:

1. In a large mixing bowl, beat butter and sour cream until blended. Add in egg yolk and mix well. Combine flour and salt and add to butter mixture. Mix well. Cover and refrigerate for at least 4 hours or overnight.

2. In a small bowl, combine the pecans or walnuts, Swerve and cinnamon.

3. Divide dough into eighths. Roll out dough, on a well-floured surface, into a 10 inch circle. Cut each circle into 8 triangles. Spread the nut mixture on top of each triangle.

4. Roll up the triangles and place point side down on parchment lined baking sheet. Bake at 350 for 15-20 minutes or until lightly brown. Let cool and sprinkle with Swerve confectioners.

No Sugar Baker's
Pumpkin Pecan Torte

Pecan Layer Ingredients:
¾ C. Swerve Brown
½ C. Butter
3 T. Heavy Whipping Cream
1 C. Chopped Pecans

Cake Ingredients:
4 Eggs
1 ⅔ C. Swerve Granular
1 C. Melted Butter OR Vegetable Oil
2 C. Canned Pumpkin Puree
½ t. Vanilla

2 C. Almond or All Purpose Flour
2 t. Baking Powder
2 t. Pumpkin Pie Spice
1 t. Baking Soda
½ t. Salt

Whipped Cream Topping Ingredients:
2 C. Heavy Whipping Cream
½ C. Swerve Confectioners
1 t. Vanilla

Easy Directions:

1. In a saucepan, combine all of the "pecan layer" ingredients, except the pecans. Bring to a slight rolling boil and pour into a well-greased 9 inch baking pan.

2. Sprinkle the pecans on top and set aside—letting cool. In a mixing bowl, beat the Swerve, sugar and butter/oil. Add in the pumpkin and vanilla.

3. Carefully, add in the rest of the ingredients. Make sure it is not over mixed but well blended.

4. Pour cake mixture on top of pecan layer. Bake at 350 for 35 minutes. Let cool. Flip the pan and the pecan layer will now be on top of your serving dish.

5. In electric mixer, whip all whipped cream topping ingredients until fluffy. Top the pecan layer/cake. Enjoy! (You can reduce the cake ingredients by ½ if you prefer a more flatter cake.)

No Sugar Baker's
Make Like a Twix

Crust Ingredients:
½ C. Sliced Almonds
1 ½ C. Almond Flour
4 T. Melted Butter
¼ C. Swerve Confectioners
¼ t. Salt

Caramel Ingredients:
½ C. Swerve Brown
5 T. Butter
¼ C. Allulose

½ C. Heavy Whipping Cream
1 t. Vanilla
½ t. Xanthan Gum
¼ t. Salt

Topping Ingredients:
2 C. Lily's Dark Chocolate Chips

Easy Directions:

1. Line a 9x9 inch baking pan with parchment paper and set aside. In a small bowl, combine the almond flour, Swerve Confectioners, sliced almonds and salt.

2. Add in melted butter and make into crumbly mixture. Press into pan and bake at 325 for 20 minutes. Set aside and let cool completely.

3. In a medium saucepan, bring to a rolling boil the Swerve brown, butter and Allulose. Boil for 5 minutes—stirring constantly. Remove from heat and add in the cream, vanilla and xanthan gum. Whisk in the salt. Return to the heat and boil for 3-4 more minutes.

4. Remove from heat and let caramel cool for at least 15 minutes. You want the caramel to be thickened, but spreadable. Pour onto the cooled crust and set pan in freezer for 3 hours, minimum.

5. After the freezing of 3 or more hours, melt the chocolate chips. Spread onto caramel bars and set in refrigerator overnight. Slice and enjoy!

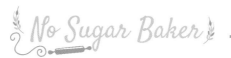
No Sugar Baker's
Chocolate Chip Cheesecake Bars

Ingredients:

1 Pkg. Keto Candy Girl Chocolate Chip Cookie Mix
½ C. Butter
3 Eggs
8 Oz. Cream Cheese
¼ C. Swerve Confectioners + 2 T.

1 C. Lily's Dark Chocolate Chips
1 t. Vanilla
Salt (A Pinch)

Easy Directions:

1. Spray a 9x9 baking dish and set aside. In a small bowl, combine the cookie mix, butter and 2 of the eggs. Mix well.

2. Spread ¾ of cookie batter in dish, keeping the ¼ remaining. In a mixing bowl, whip the cream cheese, Swerve, vanilla, 1 egg and salt.

3. Spread onto cookie batter layer. Top with remaining cookie batter and dark chocolate chips. Bake at 350 for 45 minutes. After cooled, you must refrigerate for 2-3 hours. Then, cut and serve!

No Sugar Baker's
Holy Smokes Pumpkin Bars

Bar Ingredients:
2 C. All Purpose or Almond Flour
1 ½ t. Baking Powder
1 ½ t. Baking Soda
½ t. Salt
2 t. Cinnamon
2 t. Pumpkin Pie Spice
1 C. Melted Butter OR 1 C. Vegetable Oil
3 Eggs
1 C. Swerve Brown

⅓ C. Swerve Granular
¼ C. Sugar Free Breakfast Maple Syrup
1 15 Oz. Can Pumpkin Puree
2 t. Vanilla

Cream Cheese Frosting Ingredients:
8 Oz. Cream Cheese (Room Temperature)
2 C. Swerve Confectioners
1 T. Vanilla
½ C. Heavy Whipping Cream

Easy Directions:

1. Spray a 10x15 inch baking pan and set aside. In large bowl, mix the eggs, pumpkin puree, oil or butter, vanilla, syrup, Swerve Granular and Swerve Brown.

2. In a small bowl, mix together the flour, baking soda, baking powder, spices and salt. Add to the wet ingredients mixture.

3. After combining, pour into baking dish and bake at 350 for 30-35 minutes.

4. Let cool and then refrigerate for at least 2-4 hours. You can make an easy cream cheese frosting by beating all the frosting ingredients.

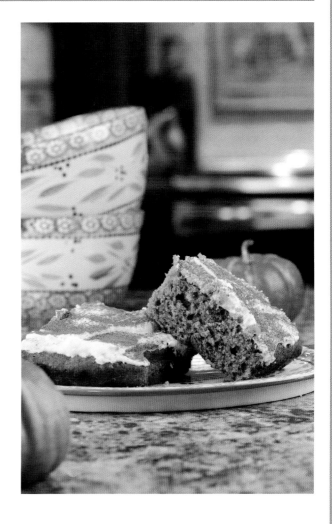

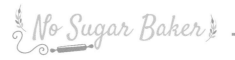
No Sugar Baker's
Chunky Monkey Cookies

Ingredients:

¾ C. Swerve Granular

¾ C. Swerve Brown

½ C. Butter

2 Eggs

1 t. Vanilla

2 T. Banana Extract

½ t. Salt

1 t. Baking Soda

2 ¼ C. Flour or Almond Flour

2 C. Lily's Dark Chocolate Chips

1 C. Chopped Walnuts

Easy Directions:

1. In a large mixing bowl, combine the Swerves, eggs, butter, vanilla and banana extract. In a small bowl, combine the flour, baking soda and salt.

2. After combined, mix the flour mixture into the wet ingredients. Add in chocolate chips and walnuts.

3. The dough will be sticky and if you prefer, you can refrigerate for 30 minutes. Spoon and drop cookie sized dough balls onto cookie baking sheet. Bake at 350 for 15-20 minutes.

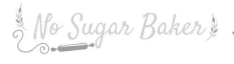
Bars, Cookies & Desserts

No Sugar Baker's
French Silk Pie

Filling Ingredients:
Make No Sugar Baker's Pie Crust Recipe or
1 Unbaked Pie Crust (Watch the Labels)
1 C. Heavy Whipping Cream
2 C. Chopped Dark Chocolate (No Sugar Added) Bars
4 Eggs
1 C. Swerve Granular

1 C. Butter
2 t. Vanilla

Topping Ingredients:
1 C. Heavy Whipping Cream
2 T. Swerve Confectioners
1 t. Vanilla

Easy Directions:

1. Bake the pie crust and let cool completely. In a large mixing bowl, whip the heavy cream until peaks form, about 5 minutes. Place in the refrigerator.

2. Melt the chocolate in a double boiler or microwave. Whisk eggs and ½ C. of Swerve in a saucepan on medium heat. You must whisk constantly until reaching a 160 degree temperature. It takes about 10 minutes.

3. Remove from heat and let cool. After cooled, stir in the melted chocolate. Let cool for another 10 minutes.

4. In a large mixing bowl, beat the butter and remaining ½ C. Swerve Granular until combined and creamy.

5. Add in the vanilla. Pour in the chocolate mixture. Continue to beat until light and fluffy. Finally add in the whipped cream. Fold until well combined. Pour into baked cooled pie crust. Refrigerate for at least 6 hours.

6. For topping, simply beat together all topping ingredients and, spread onto pie before serving.

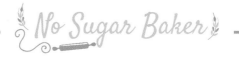
No Sugar Baker's
Dark Chocolate Pecan Pie

Ingredients:

Make No Sugar Baker's Pie Crust Recipe or Buy a Pie Crust (Watch the Labels)
3 Eggs
¾ C. Swerve Brown
1 C. Sugar Free Maple Syrup
½ C. Melted Butter
2 t. Vanilla

½ t. Salt
1 t. Cinnamon
¼ C. Sugar Free Caramel Coffee Syrup (Optional)
1 C. Lily's Dark Chocolate Chips
2 ½ C. Chopped Pecan Halves

Easy Directions:

1. Spread pecans and chocolate chips evenly over unbaked pie crust. Set aside. In a mixing bowl, whisk the eggs, Swerve, syrup, butter, vanilla, salt, and cinnamon.

2. Add in additional caramel syrup if desired. Pour mixture on top of pecans/chocolate chips.

3. Bake at 350 for 45-50 minutes. Let cool.

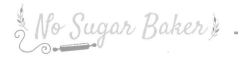

No Sugar Baker's
Lemon Raspberry Crumb Cake

Ingredients:
½ C. Butter
1 C. Swerve Granular
2 Eggs
1 C. Sour Cream
1 T. Vanilla
2 C. Almond or Regular Flour
1 t. Baking Powder
½ t. Baking Soda
½ t. Salt

¼ C. Lemon Juice
2 C. Fresh Raspberries

Topping Ingredients:
½ C. Swerve Granular
1 C. Almond or Regular Flour
½ C. Butter
1 T. Lemon Juice

Easy Directions:

1. Spray a 9 inch springform pan and line it with parchment paper. In a mixing bowl, cream butter and Swerve together. Add in eggs, sour cream, vanilla and combine.

2. In a separate small bowl, mix together flour, baking powder, baking soda and salt. Pour into wet ingredients, mix well and add lemon juice.

3. Pour into prepared pan and sprinkle all the raspberries onto top of cake, pressing them down a little.

4. In a separate small bowl, mix all topping ingredients together and pour evenly over the raspberries.

5. Bake at 350 for 60 minutes! Let cool for 15 minutes and remove from springform pan and cool completely.

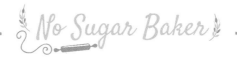

No Sugar Baker's
Pumpkin Pie Cupcakes

Ingredients:

2 C. Pumpkin Puree

½ C. Heavy Whipping Cream

2 Eggs

1 T. Vanilla

6 T. Almond Flour

1 T. Pumpkin Pie Spice

1 t. Baking Powder

½ C. Swerve Granular

½ t. Salt

Topping Ingredients:

2 T. Swerve Granular

2 T. Flour

½ t. Pumpkin Pie Spice

1 T. Heavy Whipping Cream

Easy Directions:

1. Line a muffin pan with cupcake paper liners. In a large mixing bowl, whisk together all the wet ingredients. In a small bowl, mix together all the dry ingredients.

2. Fold the dry ingredients into the wet ingredients and mix well. Fill each cupcake paper to about 95% full. In a small bowl, combine all the topping ingredients and spoon the mixture onto each cupcake.

3. Bake at 350 for 40 minutes. Cool completely in the pan and then, let cupcakes cool in refrigerator for at least an additional 3 hours.

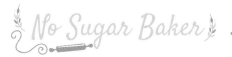

No Sugar Baker's
Dark Chocolate Pumpkin Tart

Crust Ingredients:
1 C. Flour or Almond Flour
½ C. Dark Cocoa Powder
¾ C. Swerve Granular
½ t. Salt
½ C. Butter, Melted

Filling Ingredients:
1 15 Oz. Can Pumpkin Puree
1 ½ C. Heavy Whipping Cream
1 Egg
1 T. Pumpkin Pie Spice
½ t. Salt

Easy Directions:

1. Spray a 9-inch round tart pan with a removable bottom with non-stick cooking spray and set aside. In a mixing bowl, whisk together the flour, cocoa powder, Swerve and salt. Make a well in the center and add the melted butter.

2. Stir into a crumbly dough. Press dough into the bottom and up the sides of the tart pan. Bake the crust at 425 for 10 minutes.

3. Remove and let cool while you make the filling. In a mixing bowl, whisk together the pumpkin, heavy cream, egg, pumpkin pie spice and salt. Pour onto crust.

4. Bake at 425 for 10 minutes, then reduce the temperature to 350 and bake for an additional 25-30 minutes.

5. Let cool and set in refrigerator for a few hours. You can top your tart with No Sugar Baker's whipping cream! YUM!

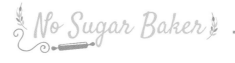

No Sugar Baker's
Pumpkin Gooey Bars

Ingredients:
2 C. Crushed Almonds OR 2 C. Graham Cracker Crumbs
½ C. Melted Butter
8 Oz. Cream Cheese
½ C. Pumpkin Puree
¼ C. Melted Butter

½ C. Swerve Brown
2 Eggs
1 T. Vanilla
½ t. Salt
1 T. Pumpkin Pie Spice
2 C. Lily's Dark Chocolate Chips
1 ½ C. Unsweetened Flaked Coconut

Easy Directions:

1. Spray an 8x8 baking pan with nonstick spray. In a small bowl, combine crushed almonds or graham cracker crumbs with melted ½ C. butter. Press into pan and set aside.

2. In large bowl, beat cream cheese until smooth, beat in pumpkin, additional ¼ C. butter, Swerve brown, eggs, vanilla, salt and pumpkin pie spice. Spread evenly over crust. Sprinkle on chocolate chips.

3. Bake at 350 for 20 minutes. Remove from oven, sprinkle coconut onto bars and bake for an additional 20 minutes.

4. Let cool. I placed my bars in refrigerator over night and the taste was superb!

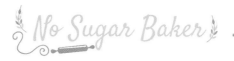
No Sugar Baker's
Pumpkin Caramel Rolls

Bread Machine Ingredients:

1 C. Unsweetened Almond Milk (Heat to 100 Degrees)

½ C. Water (About 110 Degrees—warm to the touch)

1 t. Cake Flavoring or Vanilla

½ C. Butter, Cut Into Pieces

2 Eggs (Room Temperature)

½ t. Salt

¾ C. Swerve Granular

5 C. Bread Flour (OR 3 C. Bread Flour and 2 C. Almond Flour)

3 t. Instant Active Yeast (I use Bread Machine Yeast)

Inner Roll Ingredients:

1 T. Cinnamon

4 Oz. Melted Cream Cheese

1 C. Pumpkin Puree

6 T. Melted Butter

1 T. Swerve Brown

1 T. Chopped Pecans

Cream Cheese Frosting Ingredients:

8 Oz. Cream Cheese (Room Temperature)

¾ C. Swerve Confectioners

1 T. Vanilla

2 T. Unsweetened Almond Milk

Easy Directions:

1. Put all bread machine ingredients in bread machine canister. Set on dough cycle.

2. When finished, remove dough from canister and put on lightly floured surface counter. Using rolling pin, roll out dough to ¼ inch thick. In a small mixing bowl, combine melted cream cheese, pumpkin puree and melted butter. Spread onto dough.

3. Heavily sprinkle with cinnamon and Swerve Brown. Sprinkle chopped pecans. Starting from an outside edge, rollup dough tightly like a jelly roll. In a 9x12 baking pan, grease or spray baking pan and sprinkle with Swerve brown and additional cinnamon.

4. Cut dough into 12 even pieces. Place rolls into pan. Cover with a dish towel and let rise until double in size (about one hour). Bake at 375 for 25-30 minutes.

5. Let cool for 5 minutes and remove from pan. You can make a cream cheese frosting by whipping together all the frosting ingredients and then, spread onto cooled rolls.

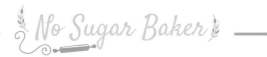

Bars, Cookies & Desserts

No Sugar Baker's
Peanut Butter Chocolate Chip Cookies

Ingredients:

2 ½ C. Flour or Almond Flour

1 t. Baking Soda

1 t. Baking Powder

½ t. Salt

½ C. Butter

¾ C. Deli Fresh Peanut Butter

½ C. Swerve Granular

1 C. Swerve Brown

2 Large Eggs + 1 Egg Yolk

2 t. Vanilla

2 C. Lily's Dark Chocolate Chips

Easy Directions:

1. In a large mixing bowl, mix butter and peanut butter until creamy. Add in both Swerves, eggs and vanilla. Mix thoroughly.

2. In a separate small bowl, combine the flour, soda, baking powder and salt. Add this mixture to the large mixing bowl and combine.

3. Finish by adding in the chocolate chips. Roll into cookie dough size balls and bake at 350 for 9-10 minutes.

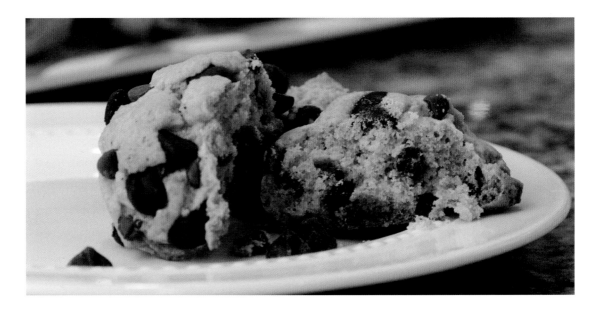

No Sugar Baker's
Pumpkin Roll

Cake Ingredients:

3 T. Swerve Confectioners

¾ C. Flour or Almond Flour

½ t. Baking Powder

½ t. Baking Soda

½ t. Cinnamon

½ t. Pumpkin Pie Spice

½ t. Salt

3 Eggs

1 C. Swerve Granular

1 15 Oz. Can Pumpkin Puree

Filling Ingredients:

8 Oz. Cream Cheese

1 C. Swerve Confectioners

6 T. Butter

1 T. Vanilla

Easy Directions:

1. For cake: Preheat oven to 375. Grease a 13x18 inch pan and line with parchment paper. You can do the same to the parchment paper to ensure it doesn't stick. Sprinkle a thin, cotton kitchen towel with 3-4 tablespoons of Swerve Confectioners.

2. Combine flour, baking powder, baking soda, spices and salt in a small bowl. Beat eggs and Swerve Granular in larger mixer bowl. Beat in pumpkin. Stir in flour mixture. Spread evenly into prepared pan.Bake at 350 for 40 minutes.

3. Immediately loosen and turn cake onto prepared towel. Peel off paper. Roll up cake and towel together, starting with narrow end.

4. For filling: Beat cream cheese, Swerve Confectioners, butter and vanilla in small mixer bowl until smooth. Carefully unroll cake; remove towel. Spread cream cheese mixture over cake. Reroll cake. Wrap in plastic wrap and refrigerate at least one hour. Sprinkle with Swerve Confectioners.

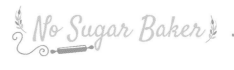

No Sugar Baker's
Autumn Spice Bundt Cake

Cake Ingredients:
1 C. Butter
2 C. Swerve Granular
4 Eggs
2 T. Vanilla
1 15 Oz. Can Pumpkin Puree
3 C. Flour or Almond Flour
2 t. Baking Powder
1 t. Baking Soda
2 T. Cinnamon

1 T. Pumpkin Pie Spice
1 t. Nutmeg

Glaze Ingredients:
½ C. Butter, Melted
1 T. Vanilla
1 T. Heavy Cream
1 C. Swerve Confectioners
Pumpkin Pie Spice to Top!

Easy Directions:

1. Spray a 10-inch (12 cup) round bundt pan. Set aside. In a large mixing bowl, beat the butter and Swerve until light and fluffy. Add eggs, vanilla and pumpkin. Mix until just combined.

2. In a separate mixing bowl, whisk together the dry ingredients--flour, baking powder, baking soda, cinnamon and pumpkin pie spice. Now, add this mixture to the liquid ingredients beating at low speed until the batter is blended.

3. Bake at 325 for 60 minutes. Cool in pan for about 15 minutes before removing from pan. Let cool completely.

4. For the simple glaze, combine all glaze ingredients in a small bowl. It will look similar to a drizzle. Pour lightly over the cake!

No Sugar Baker's Triple Berry Bars

Ingredients:

1 C. Swerve Granular

1 T. Baking Powder

3 C. Almond, Protein or All-Purpose Flour

½ t. Salt

1 C. Cold Butter

1 Egg

1 T. Vanilla

5 C. Fresh or Frozen Mixed Berries (Strawberries, Blueberries, Blackberries)

1 C. Swerve Granular

4 t. Cornstarch

½ C. Lemon Juice

Easy Directions:

1. Line a 9x13 baking pan with parchment paper and set aside. In a mixing bowl, combine Swerve, baking powder, flour, salt and cold butter. Then, add in egg and vanilla.

2. Pat half of batter into baking pan. In a separate bowl, combine berries, additional Swerve, cornstarch and lemon juice.

3. Pour mixture onto crust. Top berries with remaining crust dough evenly. Bake at 375 for 45 minutes. Let cool! Top with your favorite homemade whipped topping!

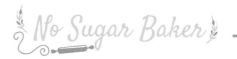
No Sugar Baker's
Vanilla Strawberry Crème Cake

Cake Ingredients:
4 C. Almond Flour
½ t. Salt
2 t. Baking Powder
1 t. Baking Soda
1 ½ C. Butter
2 C. Swerve Granular
3 Eggs + 2 Egg Whites
2 T. Vanilla
1 ½ C. Heavy Cream

Filling Ingredients:
8 Oz. Strawberry Cream Cheese
1 T. Vanilla
½ C. Butter, Melted
¾ C. Swerve Confectioners
1 C. Fresh Strawberries (Diced)

Frosting Ingredients:
1 ½ C. Butter
5 C. Swerve Confectioners
½ C. Heavy Cream
1 T. Vanilla

Easy Directions:

1. Start by greasing and preparing three 9-inch cake pans, lining with parchment paper and also spraying parchment paper. Set aside. In large bowl, whisk the flour, salt, baking powder and baking soda together. Set aside.

2. In a mixing bowl, mix butter and Swerve. When combined, add in eggs, vanilla and heavy cream. Next, add in flour mixture and mix until just combined. Pour into cake pans evenly. Bake at 350 degrees for 25 minutes. Let cool.

3. You can make the filling while the cakes are baking. In a mixing bowl, mix all filling ingredients and refrigerate until ready to assemble the cake.

4. Next, you can also pre-make the frosting. In a mixing bowl, whip all ingredients until smooth.

5. When the cake is cooled, place a small amount of filling onto serving dish. Place a cake layer on top. Spread filling over cake and place another cake layer. Repeat. When ready, frost your cake! Enjoy!!

No Sugar Baker's
Turtle Brownies

Caramel Sauce Ingredients:

6 T. Butter

¾ C. Swerve Brown

¾ C. Heavy Whipping Cream

1 t. Baking Soda

½ t. Salt

1 T. Water

Brownies Ingredients:

1 ½ C. Swerve Granular

1 C. Almond Flour

1 C. Cocoa

½ C. Swerve Confectioners

½ t. Salt

2 Eggs

½ C. Melted Butter OR ½ C. Extra Virgin Olive Oil

2 T. Water

1 T. Vanilla

2 C. Chopped Pecans

Easy Directions:

1. In a saucepan, combine the butter and Swerve Brown. Bring to a slight boil. Remove from heat, add in remaining ingredients. Return to heat and bring to a slight boil. Set aside and let cool.

2. In a mixing bowl, combine Swerve Granular, flour, cocoa, Swerve Confectioners and salt. Add in the eggs, melted butter, water and vanilla. Mix slightly until combined. Sprinkle in pecans.

3. Line an 8x8 inch baking pan with parchment paper. Pour ½ of the batter into the pan, and then spread the caramel mixture on top. Continue topping with the remaining brownie batter. Bake at 350 for 30 minutes.

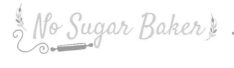
No Sugar Baker's
Blueberry Buckle

Cake Ingredients:
¾ C. Swerve Granular
½ C. Butter
1 Egg
1 T. Lemon Zest
1 ½ C Flour or Almond Flour
3 t. Baking Powder
½ t. Salt
½ C. Heavy Whipping Cream
2 C. Fresh Blueberries

Topping Ingredients:
½ C. Butter, Melted
¼ C. Swerve Brown
¼ C. Swerve Granular
¼ C. Chopped Pecans
⅓ C. Flour
1 t. Cinnamon
2 C. Chopped Pecans

Easy Directions:

1. In a large mixing bowl, cream the Swerve and butter. Add in the egg and heavy whipping cream. Mix well. Stir in the flour, baking powder and salt.

2. When combined, fold in the fresh blueberries. Pour into prepared sprayed an 8x8 baking pan. Set aside. In a small bowl, combine all the topping ingredients.

3. It will become crumbly. Sprinkle over the cake batter and bake at 350 for 45 minutes. I added a whipped topping to add extra sparkle! Enjoy!

No Sugar Baker's
Blueberry Pie Bars

Crust Ingredients:

½ C. Chilled Butter, Cut Into Cubes

¾ C. Swerve Granular

1 ½ C. Flour or Almond Flour

1 t. Cinnamon

Filling Ingredients:

1 Egg

½ C. Heavy Whipping Cream Or Sour Cream

½ C. Swerve Granular

2 T. Lemon Juice

4 t. Cornstarch

1 T. Vanilla

1 t. Cinnamon

3 C. Fresh Blueberries

Easy Directions:

1. Line an 8x8 baking pan with parchment paper. I also sprayed the parchment paper. In a food processor, combine all crust ingredients.

2. Reserve ¾ C. of the finished crust dough and set aside. Pat remaining crust down into the prepared pan. In a bowl, mix all filling ingredients besides the blueberries!

3. When mixed, fold in half of the blueberries. Pour onto crust. Top with remaining blueberries. Take the reserved dough and sprinkle it on top of the blueberries. Bake at 350 for 60 minutes.

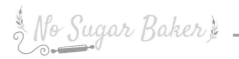
No Sugar Baker's
Blueberry Cream Cheese Coffeecake

Ingredients:

½ C. Butter

1 Egg

1 C. Heavy Whipping Cream

1 ½ C. Flour or Almond Flour

3 t. Baking Powder

½ t. Salt

1 C. Swerve Granular

4 C. Fresh Blueberries

8 Oz. Cream Cheese

Easy Directions:

1. In 8x10 baking dish, place butter. Put into oven at 350 and melt butter. In a mixing bowl, combine all ingredients but blueberries and cream cheese.

2. After butter is melted, spread butter throughout pan. Pour batter onto butter. Pat blueberries onto batter.

3. Then, place cut chunks of cream cheese throughout blueberries—making sure that every angle has cream cheese. Bake for 45 minutes. Serve warm! Watch out—this is yummy!!

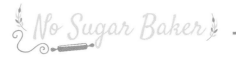

No Sugar Baker's
Strawberry Rhubarb Pie

Ingredients:

2 C. Fresh Chopped Rhubarb

3 C. Fresh Sliced Strawberries

1 C. Swerve Granular

¼ C. Flour

1 T. Cornstarch

2 T. Butter

1 Egg Yolk
(Extra Granular if You Want)

1 Prepared 9-inch Pie Double Crust (You can use the No Sugar Baker's Pie Crust Recipe)

Easy Directions:

1. In a medium mixing bowl, combine rhubarb, strawberries, Swerve Granular, flour, and corn starch. Pour into pie crust. Dab with butter.

2. Top with remaining crust. Be sure to seal the edges! Apply yolk to crust, sprinkle with a little Swerve Granular and cut small holes and pricks allowing the steam to escape.

3. Bake at 400 for 35-40 minutes. Let cool!

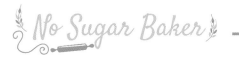
No Sugar Baker's
Ooey Gooey Butter Cake

Crust Ingredients:
1 Swerve Yellow Cake Mix
1 Egg
½ C. Butter, Melted

Filling Ingredients:
8 Oz. Cream Cheese
2 Eggs
1 T. Vanilla
½ C. Butter, Melted
3 C. Swerve Confectioners

Easy Directions:

1. In a small bowl, mix the crust ingredients and pat into a prepared sprayed 10x10 pan. In a mixing bowl, beat together the filling ingredients.

2. When combined and smooth, pour onto crust. Bake at 350 for 45-50 minutes. The center will be giggly.

3. Cool and refrigerate. Serve with whipped cream, Swerve confectioners and berries!

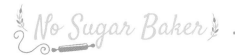

No Sugar Baker's
Strawberry Rhubarb Crumble

Ingredients:
2 C. Fresh Chopped Rhubarb
3 C. Fresh Sliced Strawberries
½ C. Swerve Granular
Zest from 1 Lemon
1 T. Lemon Juice
Salt (A Pinch)

Crumble Topping Ingredients:
¾ C. Chopped Pecans
1 C. Almond Flour
1 T. Cinnamon
½ t. Salt
½ C. Swerve Granular
½. C. Butter, Cubes

Easy Directions:

1. In a medium mixing bowl, combine rhubarb, strawberries, lemon zest, lemon juice, Swerve Granular and salt. Spread into 10x10 inch baking pan.

2. In a mixing bowl, mix pecans, almond flour, cinnamon, salt and Swerve Granular. Cut in butter. Using your hands combine the mixture – it will form crumbs like a crust.

3. Put on top of berry mixture, spreading evenly. Bake at 350 for 30 minutes. You can serve warm or cool—we like it with whipped cream!

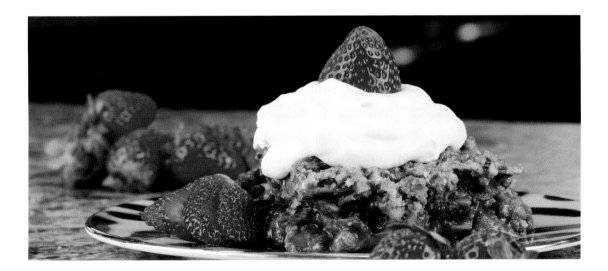

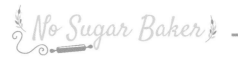

No Sugar Baker's
Double Chocolate Brownie

Bottom Layer Ingredients:
1 Swerve Chocolate Cake Mix
½ C. Butter, Melted
1 Egg

Top Layer Ingredients:
8 Oz. Cream Cheese

½ C. Butter Melted
2 Eggs
½ C. Cocoa
1 T. Vanilla
2 ¼ C. Swerve Confectioners

Easy Directions:

1. Spray a 9x9 inch baking pan and set aside. In a small bowl, mix cake mix, butter and egg. Your mixture will be thick, pat into pan and set aside.

2. In a large mixing bowl, whip cream cheese until light and fluffy. Add in butter, eggs, cocoa, vanilla and Swerve.

3. When combined and mixed well, pour onto cake layer. Bake at 350 for 50-60 minutes.

4. The brownie will appear to be jiggly. Set in the refrigerator overnight. You can sprinkle Swerve Confectioners on top!

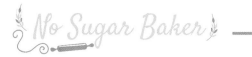
No Sugar Baker's Famous Chocolate Chip Cheesecake Cookies

Cheesecake Filling Ingredients:
4 Oz. Cream Cheese
½ C. Swerve Confectioners

1 T. Vanilla
2 C. Lily's Dark Chocolate Chips

Dough Ingredients:
2 ½ C. Flour or Almond Flour
1 t. Baking Soda
½ t. Salt
1 C. Butter
1 C. Swerve Brown
1 Egg + 1 Egg Yolk

Easy Directions:

1. In a small bowl, combine the cheesecake filling ingredients and place in the refrigerator while you make the cookie dough.

2. In a large mixing bowl, cream together butter and Swerve, and egg/egg yolk. Add in vanilla. Mix well. In a separate bowl, combine flour, soda, and salt. Add to butter mixture.

3. Fold in chocolate chips.

4. Next, take the cheesecake filling out of the refrigerator and roll filling into very small balls. Wrap each cheesecake ball with cookie dough.

5. Place on cookie baking sheet. Bake at 375 for 10-12 minutes. Let cool.

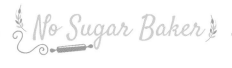
No Sugar Baker's
Fresh Strawberry Pie

Crust Ingredients:
2 C. Almond Flour
½ C. Swerve Granular
½ t. Salt
½ C. Butter, Melted

Filling Ingredients:
1 Pint Fresh Sliced Strawberries
1 C. Swerve Granular
¾ C. Water

1 T. Lemon Juice
3 T. Cornstarch
3 T. Butter

Topping Ingredients:
1 C. Heavy Whipping Cream
3 T. Cream Cheese (Room Temperature)
3 T. Swerve Confectioners
1 T. Vanilla

Easy Directions for Crust:

1. Combine all the ingredients. Pat firmly in heavily greased or sprayed pie pan. Prick the crust with a fork. Bake for 15 minutes at 325. Let cool.

Easy Directions for Pie:

1. On stovetop, bring 2 C. of sliced strawberries, water, lemon juice and cornstarch to a boil, stirring frequently. Let boil for 2 minutes, stirring constantly. Remove from heat, add in butter and stir until melted. Let cool for one hour.

2. Put remaining sliced strawberries into pie shell, pour strawberry mixture over fresh strawberries and place in refrigerator for at least 4 hours. This will allow the pie to set.

Easy Directions for Topping:

1. In a mixing bowl, combine all ingredients and whip until peaks form.
   Top your pie!

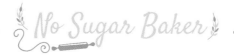

No Sugar Baker's
Coconut Cream Pie

Filling Ingredients:
2 C. Unsweetened Flake Coconut
1 ½ C. Half-and-Half or Heavy Whipping Cream
1 ½ C. Unsweetened Coconut Milk
2 Beaten Eggs
½ C. Flour
¼ t. Salt
1 t. Vanilla

Crust Ingredients:
2 C. Almond Flour
½ C. Swerve Confectioners
1 T. Cinnamon
½ t. Salt
½ C. Butter, Melted

Easy Directions:

1. First, we will prepare the crust! In dry skillet, sauté the almond flour until golden brown—about 2 minutes, stirring constantly. Mix the almond flour with the rest of the crust ingredients.

2. Press into greased pie pan, and place in freezer while you make the pie filling! In oven, at 300, toast coconut on cookie sheet until very light brown. It will be less than 5 minutes! Set aside.

3. On stovetop, in medium sized saucepan, mix half-and-half or cream, coconut milk, eggs, flour, and salt. Bring to a slow boil. Stirring constantly. Let boil for 4-5 minutes. Add in vanilla. Add in 1 ½ C. Coconut (leaving remaining for pie topping!

4. Top the pie crust with your prepared filling. Place in refrigerator for at least 5 hours. When ready to serve, whip together heavy whipping cream, Swerve Confectioners and vanilla. Top your pie with the whipped cream and remaining coconut.

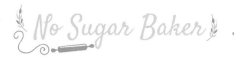

No Sugar Baker's
Strawberry Rhubarb Delightful Bars

Bar Ingredients:
2 C. Fresh or Frozen Unsweetened Rhubarb, Sliced into Small Pieces
2 C. Fresh Sliced Strawberries
½ C. Swerve Granular
1 T. Water
1 T. Lemon Juice
2 T. Cornstarch

Crust Ingredients:
1 ½ C. Almond Flour
1 C. Sliced Almonds

1 C. Swerve Brown
¾ C. Melted Butter
1 t. Baking Soda
½ t. Salt

Glaze Ingredients:
¾ C. Swerve Confectioners
2 T. Heavy Whipping Cream

Easy Directions:

1. Combine rhubarb, strawberries, water, Swerve and lemon juice in middle sized saucepan. Cook over medium heat. Bring to a boil. Stirring constantly. Let boil for 2-3 minutes. Remove from heat, add in cornstarch and mix. Let sit.

Easy Directions for Crust:

1. Combine all ingredients in a mixing bowl. Mix until mixture resembles coarse crumbs. Put 1 ½ C. crumb mixture aside. Press remaining mixture into the bottom of a greased 13x9 baking pan. Spread filling over crust. Sprinkle reserved crumb mixture on top of filling. Bake at 350 for 35-40 minutes. It will be a light golden brown.

Easy Directions for Glaze:

1. Mix the glaze ingredients and after bars have cooled, you can glaze bars with this sweet topping!

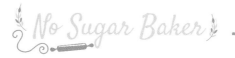

No Sugar Baker's
Give Em Chocolate Cake

Coffeecake Layer Ingredients:
3 C. Almond Flour
¾ C. Dark Chocolate Cocoa Powder
5 t. Baking Powder
½ t. Salt
¾ C. Heavy Whipping Cream
3 Eggs
¾ C. Swerve Granular
4 t. Vanilla

Filling Ingredients:
½ C. Hot Water
4 T. Dark Chocolate Cocoa Powder
2 C. Lily's Dark Chocolate Chips
2 C. Heavy Whipping Cream
2 T. Swerve Granular

Frosting Ingredients:
½ C. Dark Chocolate Cocoa Powder
8 Oz. Cream Cheese (Room Temperature)
¼ C. Butter
3 C. Swerve Confectioners
4 T. Heavy Whipping Cream
1 T. Vanilla

Easy Directions for Cake:

1. Mix all ingredients until smooth. Pour into two greased, lined with parchment paper 8-inch pans. Bake at 350 for 15-16 minutes. Let cool.

Easy Directions for Filling:

1. While the cake is baking, make this yummy filling. Stir the cocoa into the hot water. Melt the chocolate chips and add the cocoa mix. In a mixing bowl, whip on high the whipping cream and Swerve.

2. After peaks have formed, add in chocolate chips/cocoa mixture. Stir. When smooth, place in refrigerator until ready to assembly cooled cakes.

Easy Directions for Frosting:

1. Place all ingredients in a mixing bowl, mix on high until frosting is made. Now the fun part! On serving platter, put a good amount of filling onto the platter as your "glue" placing one of the cakes on top. Spread the remaining filling onto the cake, in the middle. Place second cake onto filling. Frost cake with the frosting! Enjoy!

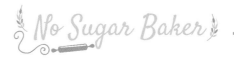
No Sugar Baker's
Chocolate Peanut Butter Dessert

Crust Ingredients:
2 C. Almond Flour
2 T. Melted Butter
4 T. Cocoa Powder
½ C. Swerve Granular

Filling Ingredients:
8 Oz. Mascarpone or Cream Cheese
1 C. Deli Fresh Peanut Butter
2 C. Heavy Whipping Cream

3 T. Vanilla
½ T. Salt
½ C. Swerve Confectioners

Topping Ingredients:
2 T. Deli Fresh Peanut Butter
2 C. Lily's Dark Chocolate Chips
1 T. Heavy Whipping Cream
½ C. Salted Peanuts

Easy Directions for Crust:

1. Mix butter, flour, cocoa and Swerve Granular. Pat into 9 inch baking pan and bake at 350 for 10 minutes. Place in freezer before moving on to the filling.

Easy Directions for Filling:

1. In a small bowl, mix the cheese and peanut butter. Set aside. In an electric mixing bowl, mix the whipping cream, vanilla, salt and Swerve until peaks forms and hold. Carefully, add in peanut butter mixture. Beat until smooth.

2. Take a taste—does it need more vanilla or salt or peanut butter—add a little until taste is delightful to you! Spread on top of crust and freeze for at least one hour.

Easy Directions for Topping:

1. Melt the peanut butter and chocolate chips. Stir in the whipping cream. Spread onto dessert and top with peanuts. Refreeze until ready to serve. You can eat frozen or let dessert thaw slightly for an hour before serving in fridge.

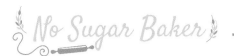

No Sugar Baker's Peanut Butter Chocolate Chip Pecan Cookies

Ingredients:

1 C. Butter

2 C. Swerve Brown

2 Eggs

4 t. Vanilla

1 C. Deli Fresh Peanut Butter

1 ½ C. Flour

1 ¼ C. Almond Flour

3 t. Baking Soda

½ t. Salt

2 C. Lily's Dark Chocolate Chips

1 ½ C. Chopped Pecans

Easy Directions:

1. In a mixing bowl, combine butter and Swerve. Add eggs, vanilla, and peanut butter and mix again. In a separate small bowl, combine flours, soda and salt.

2. Add flour mixture to first mixture and combine well. Add in chocolate chips and pecans. The dough will be more firm than other cookie doughs. Make round balls and place on sprayed cookie sheet. Bake at 375 for 12-14 minutes, until light golden brown.

3. They will look like mounds—that's a good sign! Take out of oven and carefully flatten each cookie until desired thickness with the back of a spatula. Let cool.

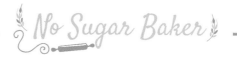

No Sugar Baker's Cinnamon Pie

Crust Ingredients:
2 C. Almond Flour
½ C. Swerve Granular
½ t. Salt
½ C. Melted Butter

Filling Ingredients:
1 C. Swerve Brown
1 ½ C. Heavy Whipping Cream

8 Oz. Cream Cheese
2 Eggs + 1 Egg Yolk
¼ C. Flour (You can use almond or coconut flour)
4 T. Cinnamon
3 t. Vanilla
½ t. Salt
1 t. Nutmeg

Easy Directions:

1. In a small bowl, combine almond flour, Swerve Granular, salt and butter to make the crust. Pat into pie pan and bake at 350 for 10 minutes. Set aside and let cool.

2. In a mixing bowl, beat cream cheese and Swerve together until light and creamy. Beat in the eggs. Add in cream, flour, cinnamon, vanilla, salt and nutmeg. Mix until smooth and silky.

3. Pour on top of crust prepared pie pan. Bake at 350 for 40-45 minutes. Let cool and place in refrigerator. I let our pie rest in fridge overnight.

4. I also topped our slices with homemade whipping cream. I used my electric mixer and whipped together heavy whipping cream (approximately 1 C.), vanilla (1 T.) and Swerve Confectioners (1/2 C.).

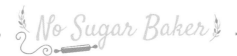

Michael Del Zotto's
Protein No Sugar Carrot Cake

Cake Ingredients:
2 ½ C. Almond Flour
3 t. Baking Powder
3 t. Cinnamon
1 t. Nutmeg
½ t. Salt
1 C. Swerve Granular
½ C. Butter
½ C. Unsweetened Applesauce
4 Eggs
¼ C. Heavy Whipping Cream

1 T. Vanilla
2 C. Shredded Organic Carrots (Pureed)
2 C. Chopped Pecans

Cream Cheese Frosting Ingredients:
8 Oz. Whipped Cream Cheese
(Room Temperature)
¼ C. Heavy Whipping Cream
1 T. Vanilla
½ C. Swerve Confectioners

Easy Directions for Cake:

1. In a small bowl, combine the flour, baking powder, cinnamon, nutmeg and salt. Set aside. In a mixing bowl, combine Swerve and butter (applesauce) until smooth. Add in eggs, two at a time. Continue to mix, add in cream and vanilla. Mix again.

2. Pour in flour mixture. Combine. Add in shredded carrots. Mix. Add in pecans.

3. Mix. Pour into prepared sprayed pans (you can use two 9 inch round cake pans, a springform pan or a 10 inch square pan). Bake at 350 for 35-40 minutes. Let cool. Store in refrigerator.

Easy Directions for Frosting:

1. Combine all ingredients in mixer. Mix on high until peaks form. Spread onto layers of carrot cake or spread onto top of single layered cake.

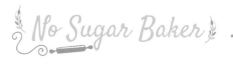
No Sugar Baker's Strawberry Cream Pie

Crust Ingredients:
2 C. Almond Flour
½ C. Swerve Granular
½ t. Salt
½ C. Melted Butter

Filling Ingredients:
1 Pint Fresh Strawberries, Sliced.
½ C. Swerve Confectioners

¼ C. Swerve Granular
8 Oz. Strawberry Cream Cheese, Softened.
1 C. Heavy Whipping Cream

Whipped Cream Topping Ingredients:
1 ½ C. Heavy Whipping Cream
½ C. Swerve Confectioners
½ t. Vanilla

Easy Directions for Crust:

1. Combine all the ingredients. Press firmly in heavily greased or sprayed pie pan. Prick the top with a fork. Bake for 15 minutes at 325. Let cool.

Easy Directions for Filling:

1. Combine all ingredients in food processor and blend. Add in heavy whipping cream and blend again until smooth. Pour onto pie crust and refrigerate overnight.

Easy Directions for Topping:

1. Combine all ingredients in mixer, mix on high until peaks form. Top the dessert with this yummy topping.

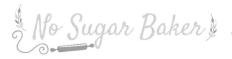

No Sugar Baker's
Lemon Blueberry Cheesecake

Crust Ingredients:
2 C. Almond Flour
½ C. Sliced Almonds
½ C. Swerve Granular
½ t. Salt
½ C. Butter, Melted.

Filling Ingredients:
32 Oz. Cream Cheese

1 C. Swerve Granular
3 T. Flour (I admit to using all-purpose flour, but almond or coconut flour can be used)
1 C. Sour Cream
¼ C. Lemon Juice
3 Eggs
3 Egg Yolks
1 Pint Fresh Blueberries
¼ C. Heavy Whipping Cream

Easy Directions for Crust:

1. Combine all the ingredients. Press firmly in heavily greased or sprayed springform pan or round pan. Prick the top with a fork. Bake for 15 minutes at 325. Let cool.

Easy Directions for Filling:

1. In a mixing bowl, combine the cream cheese and Swerve. Add in the flour and combine. Add in the sour cream, heavy whipping cream and lemon juice, combining until smooth. Add in one egg at a time, while continuing to mix. Do the same with the egg yolks. Fold in blueberries.

2. Pour mixture onto crust. Set aside. On a baking sheet or larger baking pan, fill the pan with a water bath, about enough water to cover halfway up of the cheesecake pan. Place the cheesecake pan into the water bath pan. Bake at 300 for 85 minutes. Do not open the oven! Set a timer and let it be! After the initial 85 minutes, turn off the oven and the leave the oven door closed for an additional 30 minutes. Set a timer and let it be.

3. After 30 minutes, crack the oven door slightly. And, let the cheesecake rest again for another 30 minutes. Set a timer and let it be. Remove the cheesecake and place just the cheesecake pan in the refrigerator for at least 3 hours.

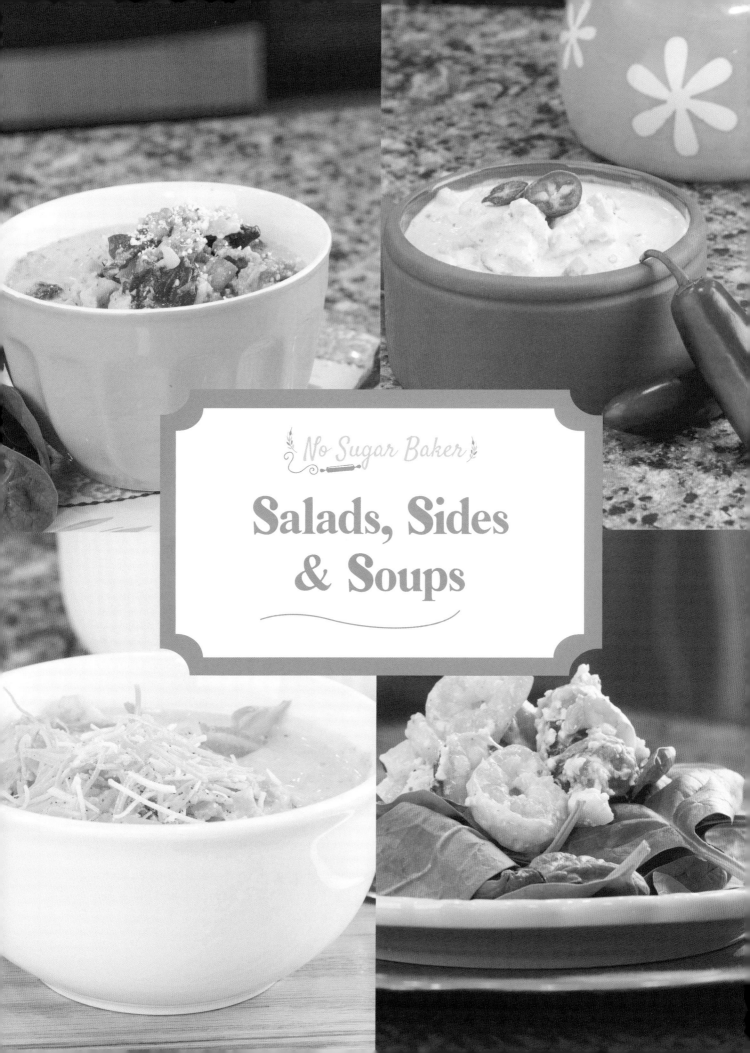

No Sugar Baker

Salads, Sides & Soups

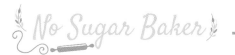
No Sugar Baker's
Cheesy Green Beans and Bacon

Ingredients:

Dash of Olive Oil

3 C. Green Beans

2 C. Crumbled Cooked Bacon

2 C. Your Choice of Cheese

Easy Directions:

1. In a large skillet, pour a little olive oil and begin to fry/cook green beans until tender.

2. Do not drain. When cooked to your preference, add in bacon and top with cheese.

3. Allow to melt. Isn't it easy and the best?!

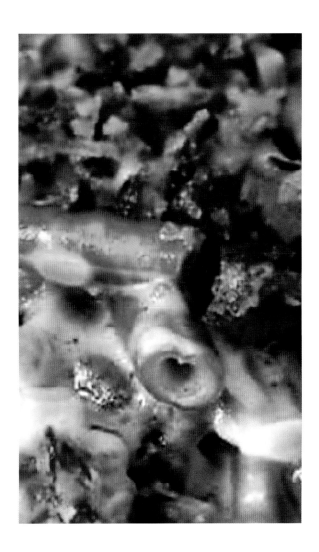

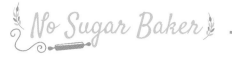

Margaret's Cranberry Sauce

Salads, Sides & Soups

Ingredients:
12 Oz. Fresh Cranberries
1 C. Swerve Confectioners
¾ C. Water
1 t. Orange Zest
1 t. Vanilla

Easy Directions:

1. In a saucepan, combine cranberries, Swerve, water and orange zest.

2. Bring to a boil and reduce heat. Let simmer for 12 minutes.

3. Remove from heat, stir in the vanilla. Let chill.

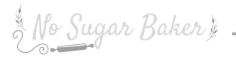

No Sugar Baker's
Hot Buns

Ingredients:

2 T. Butter

3 T. Swerve Granular

1 C. Hot Water (About 110 Degrees)

2 T. Dry Active Yeast

1 Egg

½ t. Salt

2 ¼ C. All Purpose Flour

Easy Directions:

1. In a large bowl, mix the butter, Swerve and hot water.

2. Mix in the yeast until dissolved. Add in the egg, salt and flour. Mix well.

3. Allow the dough to rise until doubled in size. Grease 8 muffin cups.

4. Divide the dough into the muffin tins and allow to rise again until double in size. (When rising, cover the dough with a towel).

5. Bake at 425 for 10 minutes.

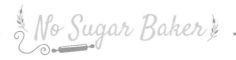
No Sugar Baker's
White Chicken Chili

Ingredients:

3 Large Cooked, Skinless Chicken Breasts
(Chopped or Shredded)

3 C. Chicken Broth

2 T. Minced Garlic

1 Can Chopped Green Chiles

1 Can Diced Jalapenos

1 C. Diced Green Peppers

½ C. Chopped Onion

4 T. Butter

½ C. Heavy Whipping Cream

8 Oz. Cream Cheese

2 t. Cumin

1 t. Oregano

1 t. Cayenne Pepper

Easy Directions:

1. In large soup pan, melt butter. Add in all spices, onion, peppers and green chiles.

2. Sauté. Add in chicken broth and cooked chicken, bring to a rolling boil.

3. In small microwavable bowl, melt cream cheese and when finished add in whipping cream.

4. Stir until well combined. Add cream cheese mixture to soup and mix thoroughly.

5. Serve with your favorite toppings—cheese, sour cream, avocado and much more!.

No Sugar Baker's
Broccoli Cheddar Soup

Ingredients:

½ C. Butter

½ C. Chopped Onion

4 C. Fresh Broccoli Florets

3 C. Chicken Broth

2 C. Heavy Cream

½ t. Salt

¼ t. Nutmeg

1 t. Pepper

¼ C. Cornstarch

3 C. Shredded Cheddar Cheese

1 C. Sour Cream

Easy Directions:

1. In Dutch oven pot, combine butter and onions.

2. Add in broccoli and chicken broth. Bring to a rolling boil for 10 minutes.

3. Reduce heat and add in cream, salt, nutmeg, pepper, cornstarch, cheese and sour cream. Mix thoroughly. Enjoy!

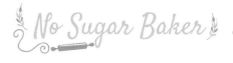

No Sugar Baker's
Spicy Taco Soup

Ingredients:

2 Lbs. Skinless, Boneless Chicken Breasts

1 C. Diced Onion

2 T. Minced Garlic

1 T. Cumin

1 T. Chili Powder

1 T. Paprika

1 T. Salt

½ C. Lemon Juice

3 C. Diced Green and Red Peppers

1 C. Sliced Jalapeno Peppers

2 C. Chicken Broth

8 Oz. Jalapeno Cream Cheese

8 Oz. Cream Cheese

2 C. Shredded Cheese

Sour Cream and Guacamole to Top!

Easy Directions:

1. In slow cooker, place chicken breasts, onion, garlic, cumin, chili powder, paprika, salt, lemon juice, all peppers and chicken broth. Cook on low for 3-4 hours.

2. When the chicken is at tender, remove it from the slow cooker and cut it into bit sized pieces and then return to slow cooker.

3. Add in cream cheeses and cheese—stir until melted.

4. When temperature at your appropriate tasting, serve in soup bowls topping with sour cream, guacamole, and more cheese!

No Sugar Baker's
Sausage Spinach Soup

Ingredients:

2 Lbs. Ground Italian Sausage

6 Slices Bacon

½ C. Chopped Onion

1 T. Butter

3 t. Minced Garlic

1 C. Chopped Green and Red Peppers

1 C. Chopped Cauliflower

64 Oz. Chicken Broth

1 ½ C. Heavy Whipping Cream

2 C. Shredded Fresh Parmesan Cheese

2 C. Fresh Spinach

Salt and Pepper to Taste

Easy Directions:

1. On stovetop in soup pot, cook the sausage and bacon. Crumble. Drain.

2. Return the meat mixture, with the butter, onion and garlic to the pot. Sauté for 1-2 minutes. Add the peppers, cauliflower and chicken broth.

3. Bring to a boil and let boil for 7-8 minutes (until the cauliflower is soft).

4. Reduce heat to a simmer, add in the cream and stir until smooth. Add in the parmesan cheese and combine.

5. Add in the spinach and stir. Enjoy!! You can top your bowl of soup with additional parmesan cheese!!

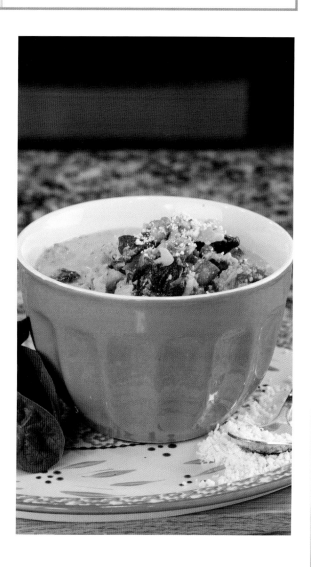

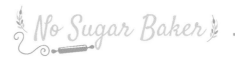

No Sugar Baker's
Jalapeno Popper Soup

Ingredients:

1 Pkg. Bacon (Cooked and Crumbled)
3 C. Chicken (Cooked and Diced)
1 T. Butter
6 Fresh Chopped Jalapeno Peppers
(Deseeded)
2 C. Chopped Green and Red Peppers
½ C. Chopped Onion

1 T. Minced Garlic
2 C. Heavy Whipping Cream
8 Oz. Jalapeno Cream Cheese
8 Oz. Cream Cheese
4 C. Shredded Cheddar Cheese
3 C. Chicken Broth
Salt to Taste

Easy Directions:

1. In Dutch oven or large pot, melt butter and add all peppers and onions. Sauté for 3 minutes.

2. Add in garlic, cream cheeses, and cream, melt the cheeses until the mixture is smooth.

3. Then, reduce heat and add in cheddar cheese, stirring until melted and smooth.

4. Add in chicken broth, stir until combined and warm. Fold in bacon and chicken.

5. Combine, salt to taste and serve in your favorite bowl!

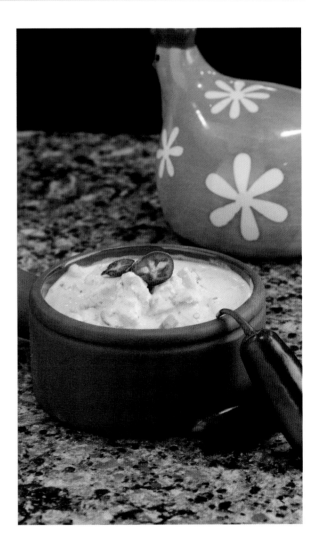

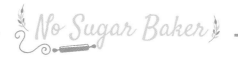
Salads, Sides & Soups

The No Sugar Baker's
Wonderful Cheeseburger Soup

Ingredients:

1 Lb. Ground Beef

4 T. Butter, Divided

¾ C. Chopped Onion

½ C. Shredded Organic Non-Orange
Colored Carrots

¾ C. Diced Celery

¾ C. Chopped Green and Yellow Peppers

1 Chopped Sweet Potato (if you prefer)

1 t. Dried Basil

1 t. Dried Parsley Flakes

2 t. Salt and Pepper

4 C. Chicken Broth

4 C. Velveeta, Cubed

1 ¼ C. Heavy Whipping Cream

½ C. Sour Cream

2 T. Flour

Easy Directions:

1. Brown the beef in large saucepan, adding the onion. Remove and drain the grease.

2. Add all vegetables to saucepan, chicken broth, and all seasonings. Bring to a boil and continue to boil for 8 minutes.

3. Reduce heat and add Velveeta cheese. Stir until fully creamed and melted. Melt butter and mix with flour.

4. Pour mixture into soup. Add heavy whipping cream and sour cream. Continue to stir and combine.

5. The soup should be at a low simmer until your appropriate eating temperature. Serve and enjoy!

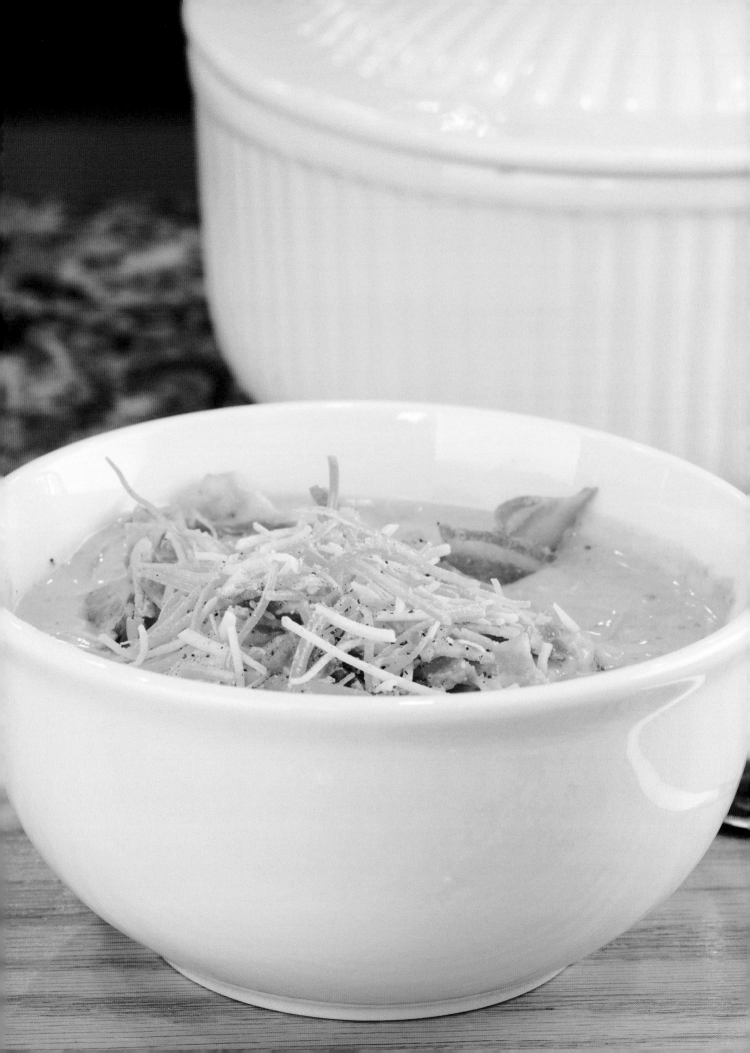

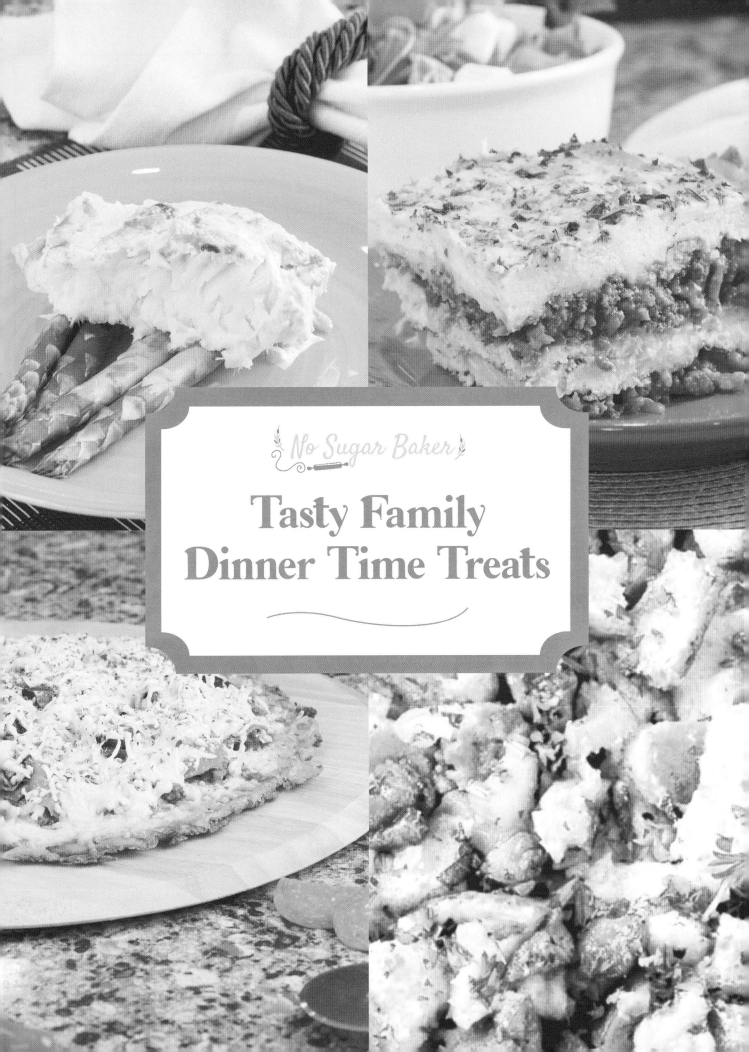

Tasty Family Dinner Time Treats

No Sugar Baker

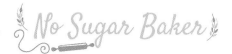
Tasty Family Dinner Time Treats

The Hub's
Sausage Stuffing

Ingredients:

1 Lb. Mild Sausage (Cooked and rumbled)

½ C. Butter

1 C. Chopped Onion

1 C. Chopped Celery

2 t. Minced Garlic

3 C. Stale Bread Crumbs (Sugar Free)

2 C. Fresh Mushrooms

2 ½ C. Chicken Broth

2 Eggs

1 T. Minced Sage Leaves

¼ C. Parsley

Easy Directions:

1. Spray an 8x10 baking dish. In a saucepan, combine the butter, sausage, mushrooms, onion and celery.

2. Cook until tender. Add garlic and cook for 30 seconds. Place the bread crumbs into a large bowl.

3. Add in the sausage mixture, chicken broth, eggs, sage, parsley, salt and pepper. Stir.

4. Spread into baking dish. Bake at 350 for 60 minutes!

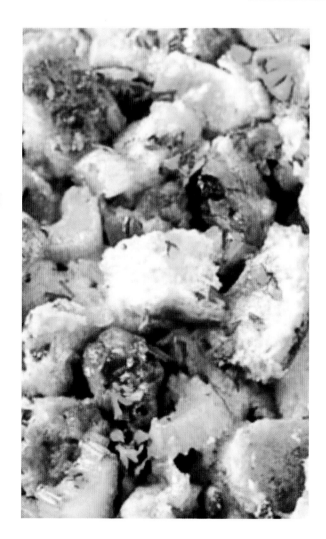

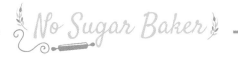

No Sugar Baker's
Chicken Bacon Ranch Pizza

Fathead Pizza Dough Ingredients:
¾ C. Almond Flour
1 ½ C. Shredded Mozzarella
2 T. Cream Cheese
1 Egg

Topping Ingredients:
2 Cooked and Sliced Skinless Boneless Chicken Breasts
6 Strips Cooked Bacon
2 C. Mozzarella Cheese
1 C. Fresh Mushrooms
1 C. Fresh Cut Green and Yellow Peppers
Ranch Dressing

Directions for Pizza Dough:

1. Melt the mozzarella and cream cheese in the microwave. Combine and stir until smooth.

2. Add almond flour and beaten egg. Combine into dough ball. Refrigerate for at least one hour.

3. Using parchment paper, roll out dough to desired thickness. Place dough on sprayed baking sheet.

4. Prick dough with fork. Bake at 400 for 10 minutes. Flip dough and repeat.

Directions:

1. Spread all toppings including Ranch dressing onto crust and finish by topping with mozzarella cheese.

2. Bake for another 10-12 minutes. Let stand for 5 minutes. Cut and enjoy!

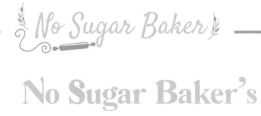

No Sugar Baker's
Chicken Alfredo Hotdish

Tasty Family Dinner Time Treats

Ingredients:

3 Cooked Skinless Boneless Chicken
Breasts, Diced

2 T. Butter

1 T. Garlic

1 T. Italian Seasonings

1 T. Parsley

½ C. Chopped Onions or Leeks

2 C. Chopped Fresh Mushrooms

1 ½ C. Heavy Whipping Cream

8 Oz. Cream Cheese

1 ½ C. Shredded Cheese of Your Choice

Easy Directions:

1. Spray a 10x12 baking dish. Put chicken into pan and set aside.

2. In a large saucepan, melt the butter. Add in garlic, Italian seasonings, onions and mushrooms.

3. Sauté until tender. Pour in cream and cream cheese, bring to a rolling boil and let thicken.

4. Pour over chicken. Add shredded cheese and bake at 350 for 30-40 minutes!

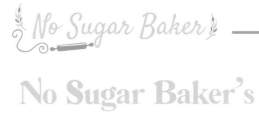

No Sugar Baker's
Chicken Enchiladas

Ingredients:

2 Skinless Boneless Chicken Breasts
1 Can Cream of Chicken Soup
1 C. Sour Cream
2 C. Chopped Mixed Fresh Peppers
2 C. Shredded Mexican Cheese
4 Egg Wraps (Found in Deli Section)

Easy Directions:

1. In large frying pan/skillet, cook chicken. Drain any excess fat. In a small bowl, combine soup and sour cream.

2. When chicken is cooked, add two large spoonfulls of soup mixture to chicken, add in all peppers and combine.

3. In an 8x8 inch baking pan, spread just enough of the soup mixture to lightly coat the bottom of the pan.

4. Now, carefully (they are very thin) take one egg wrap and spread a layer of cheese, then add a generous ¼ C. of the chicken/soup mixture, top with some more cheese. Fold it like a tortilla and place in pan.

5. Continue with the remaining egg wraps. Top all folded egg wraps with remaining soup mixture and generous amount of shredded cheese.

6. Bake at 375 for 20-25 minutes. Let sit for 5 minutes—enjoy!!

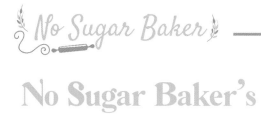

No Sugar Baker's
Chicken Like KFC

Ingredients:

5-6 Skinless Chicken Thighs, Breasts or
Legs
3 C. Crushed Pork Rinds
1 T. Black Pepper
1 T. Onion Powder
1 T. Garlic Powder

1 T. Paprika
1 T. Thyme
½ C. Mayonnaise
2 Beaten Eggs
½ C. Mustard
¼ C. Heavy Whipping Cream

Easy Directions:

1. Spray a 9x12 baking pan. In a small bowl, combine the cream, mayonnaise, eggs and mustard until smooth.

2. In a larger bowl, combine the pork rinds crumbs, pepper, powders, paprika and thyme.

3. Dip the chicken, a piece at a time, into the egg mixture and immediately coat with the pork rinds mixture.

4. Place chicken on baking pan. Bake at 400 degrees for 40-45 minutes..

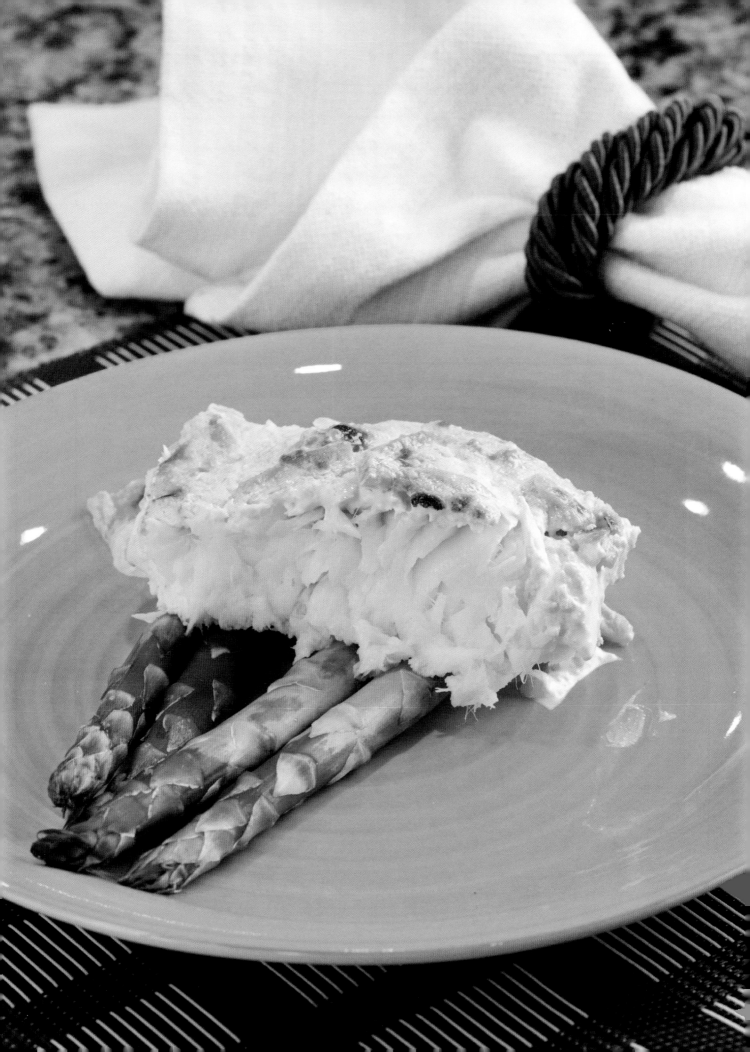

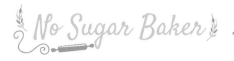

No Sugar Baker's Cheesy Saucy Halibut Or Whitefish

Ingredients:

Halibut or Whitefish Filets
1 C. Grated Parmesan Cheese
½ C. Butter
6 T. Mayonnaise
4 T. Lemon Juice
4 T. Hot Sauce

½ C. Chopped Onion
½ C. Chopped Green and Red Peppers
Dash of Salt

Easy Directions:

1. Spray a 10x10 baking dish, salt and pepper the fish filets. Bake at 400 for 10 minutes.

2. In a mixing bowl, combine all ingredients (but the fish).

3. Spread mixture on top of baked, flakey fish.

4. Bake for 10 more minutes. Broil on low for 2-4 minutes. Serve!

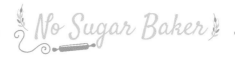
No Sugar Baker's Fresh Veggie Pizza

Dough Ingredients:
1 ¾ C. Almond Flour
½ C. Low Carbohydrate Pasta Sauce
½ t. Xanthun Gum or Corn Starch
1 t. Baking Powder
2 Eggs
1 T. Melted Butter
Splash of Seasonings: Salt, Garlic Powder, Italian Seasonings, Onion Powder

Topping Ingredients:
Sliced Vegetables of your Choice (I used: Zucchini, Asparagus, Mushrooms, Green and Red Peppers, Onions)
1 C. Low Carbohydrate Pasta Sauce
2 C. Mozzarella Cheese
Fresh Arugula or Basil
Pesto
Olive Oil

Directions for Pizza Dough:

1. Combine all ingredients in food processer into dough ball. Refrigerate for at least one hour.

2. Using parchment paper, roll out dough to desired thickness. Place dough on sprayed baking sheet.

3. Prick dough with fork. Bake at 400 for 10 minutes. Flip dough and repeat.

Directions:

1. Spread pasta sauce onto crust. Top with all your chosen vegetable toppings! Finish by topping with mozzarella cheese.

2. Bake for another 10-12 minutes. Let stand for 5 minutes.

3. Add fresh arugula or basil to the top of the pizza, along with a small scoop of pesto. You can finish it off with a light glaze of olive oil.

4. Cut and enjoy!

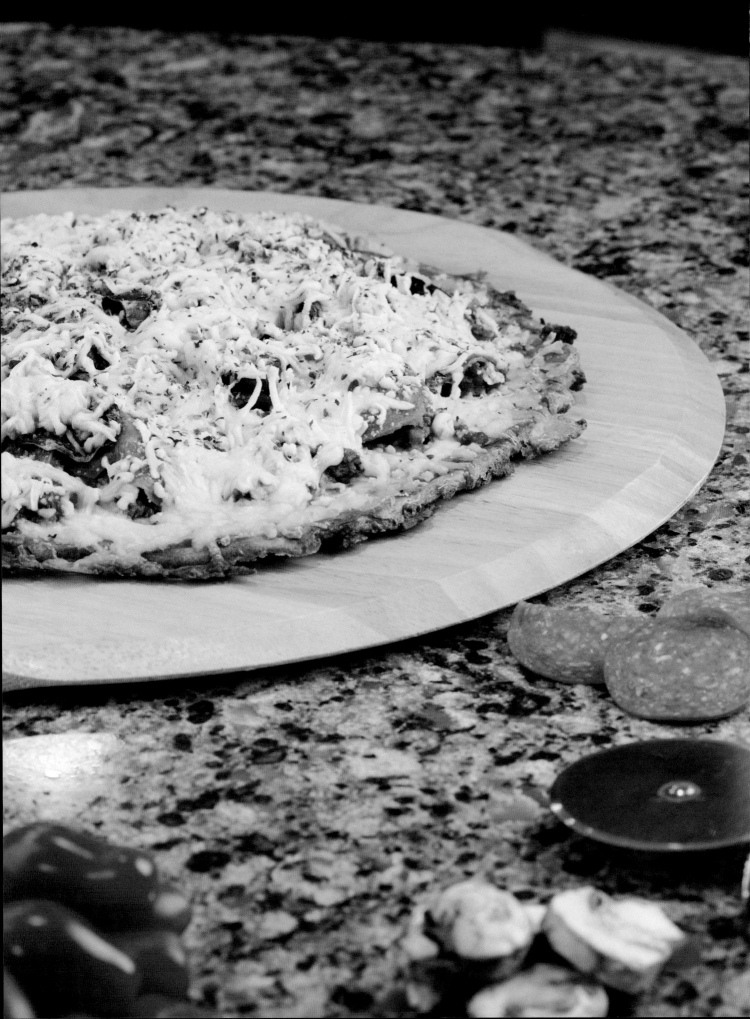

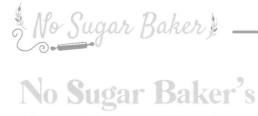
No Sugar Baker's
Air Fryer Turkey

Ingredients:

10 Lbs. or less sized Turkey
Salt and Pepper to Season
½ C. Butter (Cut into Pads)

Easy Directions:

1. Be sure to thaw your turkey in the refrigerator for two days prior to cooking. To prepare the turkey, be sure to remove the giblet bag.

2. Rinse the turkey with cold water and pat it dry. Put your fingers under the skin starting with the neck area, carefully lifting the skin and place one stick of butter pads (cubes) scattered throughout under the skin.

3. Season plentiful with salt and pepper. Place in air fryer, breast side down. Air fry at 350 for 60 minutes.

4. After the first 60 minutes, flip the turkey over with the breast side now up.

5. Continue to roast at 350 for an additional hour until the internal temperature reaches 165F.

6. Before carving, let the turkey rest. The juices may be used to make traditional turkey dressing.

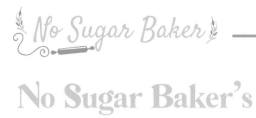

No Sugar Baker's
Sausage and Broccoli Pizza

Pizza Dough Ingredients:
1 ¾ C. Almond Flour
½ C. Low Carbohydrate Pasta Sauce
½ t. Xanthun Gum or Corn Starch
1 t. Baking Powder
2 Eggs
1 T. Melted Butter
Splash of Seasonings: Salt, Garlic Powder, Italian Seasonings, Onion Powder

Topping Ingredients:
1 Lb. Cooked Bulk Sausage
2 C. Fresh Broccoli
1 C. Low Carbohydrate Pasta Sauce
2 C. Mozzarella Cheese
Fresh Arugula or Basil
Olive Oil

Directions for Pizza Dough:

1. Combine all ingredients in food processer into dough ball. Refrigerate for at least one hour.

2. Using parchment paper, roll out dough to desired thickness. Place dough on sprayed baking sheet.

3. Prick dough with fork. Bake at 400 for 10 minutes. Flip dough over and repeat.

Directions:

1. Spread pasta sauce onto crust. Top crust with sausage and broccoli!

2. Finish by topping with mozzarella cheese. Bake for another 10-12 minutes. Let stand for 5 minutes.

3. Add fresh arugula or basil to the top of the pizza, along with a small scoop of pesto. You can finish it off with a light glaze of olive oil.

4. Cut and enjoy!

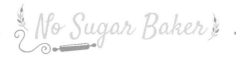

No Sugar Baker's Meat Lovers Pizza

Pizza Dough Ingredients:
2 Eggs
2 T. Sour Cream
2 T. Melted Butter
1 C. Almond Flour
1 t. Garlic Powder
Salt (A Pinch)
1 C. Shredded Cheese of Your Choice
(I prefer Cheddar or Mozzarella)

Topping Ingredients:
½ Lb. Cooked Bulk Sausage
25 Slices of Pepperoni
½ Lb. Cooked Ground Beef
3 Slices Cooked Bacon
Mushrooms
Onions
1 C. Low Carbohydrate Pasta Sauce
2 C. Mozzarella Cheese
Fresh Arugula or Basil
Olive Oil

Directions for Pizza Dough:

1. Combine all ingredients in food processer into dough ball. Refrigerate for at least one hour.

2. Using parchment paper, roll out dough to desired thickness. Place dough on sprayed baking sheet.

3. Prick dough with fork. Bake at 400 for 10 minutes. Flip dough over and repeat.

Directions:

1. Spread pasta sauce onto crust. Top crust with sausage, pepperoni, ground beef, bacon, onions and mushrooms. Finish by topping with mozzarella cheese.

2. Bake for another 10-12 minutes. Let stand for 5 minutes.

3. Cut fresh arugula or basil to the top, along with a small scoop of pesto and lightly add a glaze of olive oil! Cut and enjoy!

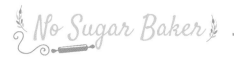

No Sugar Baker's Sloppy Joe Cornbread Casserole

Ingredients:

Make your favorite sloppy joe recipe. I used AlternaSweets BBQ Sauce and Ketchup for mine!
2 C. Shredded Cheese
1 C. Shredded Mozzarella Cheese
2 C. Almond Flour

2 Oz. Cream Cheese
3 Eggs
1 T. Baking Powder
½ t. Sweet Corn Extract

Easy Directions:

1. This is super easy.

2. Spray a cast iron skillet.

3. Make your sloppy joe recipe, mix in 1 C. of shredded cheese and set aside.

4. In a food processor, combine mozzarella cheese, cream cheese, almond flour, eggs, baking powder and corn extract. When thick like a batter, spoon into cast iron. Pour sloppy joe mixture on top and top with remaining shredded cheese. Bake for 45 minutes at 350.

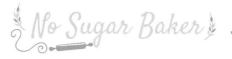

No Sugar Baker's Sloppy Fake Mac and Cheese

Ingredients:

4 C. Chopped Fresh Cauliflower
1 ½ C. Heavy Whipping Cream
8 Oz. Cream Cheese
2 C. Shredded Cheese of Your Choice
4 Slices Cooked Bacon, Diced
1 C. Pork Rinds Crumbs

Easy Directions:

1. In large saucepan, bring a pan of water to a rolling boil.

2. Add in cauliflower and boil for 7 minutes. Drain and set aside.

3. In same saucepan, pour cream, cream cheese and any additional spices you choose. After all is melted and combined, add 1 ½ C. of the shredded cheese and cauliflower.

4. Pour into pan, top with bacon, remaining cheese and pork rinds. Bake at 350 for 45 minutes.

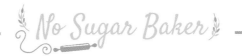
No Sugar Baker's
Spinach Parmesan Shrimp

Ingredients:

2 T. Olive Oil

3 T. Butter

2 Lbs. Deveined and Tails Removed Shrimp (Frozen or Fresh)

3 T. Garlic

1 ½ C. Grape Tomatoes

4 C. Fresh Spinach

1 C. Heavy Whipping Cream

½ C. Parmesan

3 T. Fresh Chopped Basil

Salt and Pepper to Taste

Easy Directions:

1. In large skillet, heat oil and butter until melted. Add the shrimp, toss in salt and pepper to taste and sauté for 2-3 minutes.

2. Remove shrimp from skillet and set aside. In skillet, put garlic, tomatoes, spinach and continue to sauté for 2 minutes.

3. Add in the cream, cheese and basil. Simmer for about 5 minutes stirring constantly—toss in the shrimp. Enjoy!

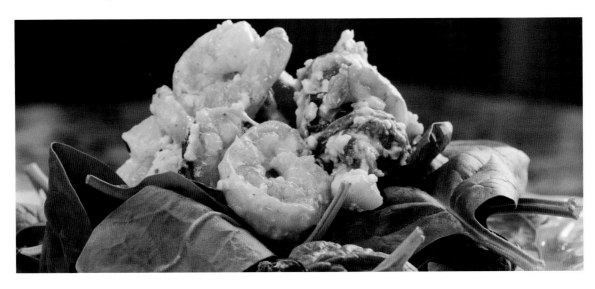

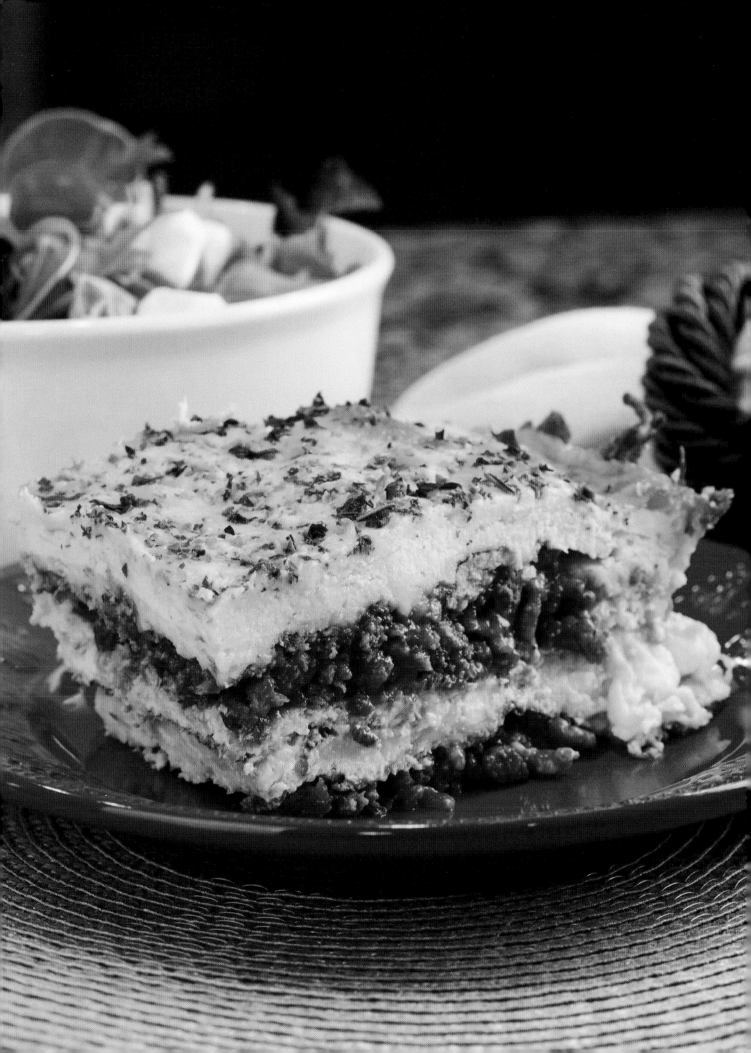

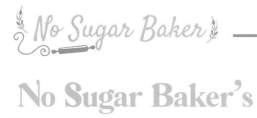

No Sugar Baker's
Zero Pasta Lasagna

Noodle Ingredients:
8 Oz. Cream Cheese
3 C. Shredded Mozzarella Cheese
4 Eggs
2 t. Italian Seasoning

Filling Ingredients:
½ C. Chopped Onion
1 Lb. Ground Beef

1 Lb. Italian Sausage
1 Jar Low Carbohydrate Pasta Sauce
1 C. Cottage Cheese
½ C. Parmesan Cheese
2 C. Shredded Mozzarella Cheese

Easy Directions:

1. Preheat oven to 350. Line two 9x13-inch baking pans with parchment paper. Melt the mozzarella and cream cheeses together. Stir until smooth and add in beaten eggs and Italian seasoning. Blend until evenly mixed. It should have a thick liquid consistency. Pour cheese batter into prepared baking pans. Use a spatula to spread batter across pans. Bake for 20 minutes. Set cheese noodles aside to let cool.

2. While noodles are cooling, prepare your meat sauce. In a large skillet, add onion, ground beef and Italian sausage. Cook on medium heat until meat is browned. Drain excess fat from pan. Add in Italian seasoning and pasta sauce.

3. Reduce to low heat and cook at a simmer. Next, evenly slice your cheese dough into thirds. Add a thin layer of meat sauce to the bottom of the pan. Add first noodle layer over meat sauce. Mix the cottage cheese with the parmesan cheese. Add 1/2 of the remaining meat sauce across first noodle layer. Spread an even layer of the cottage cheese mixture across the noodle layers. Repeat with second noodle, meat sauce, cottage cheese mixture, and mozzarella. Add third noodle. Top with remaining meat sauce. Sprinkle on remaining mozzarella. Bake lasagna at 350 for about 30 minutes. Let lasagna set for 5 minutes. Serve and enjoy!

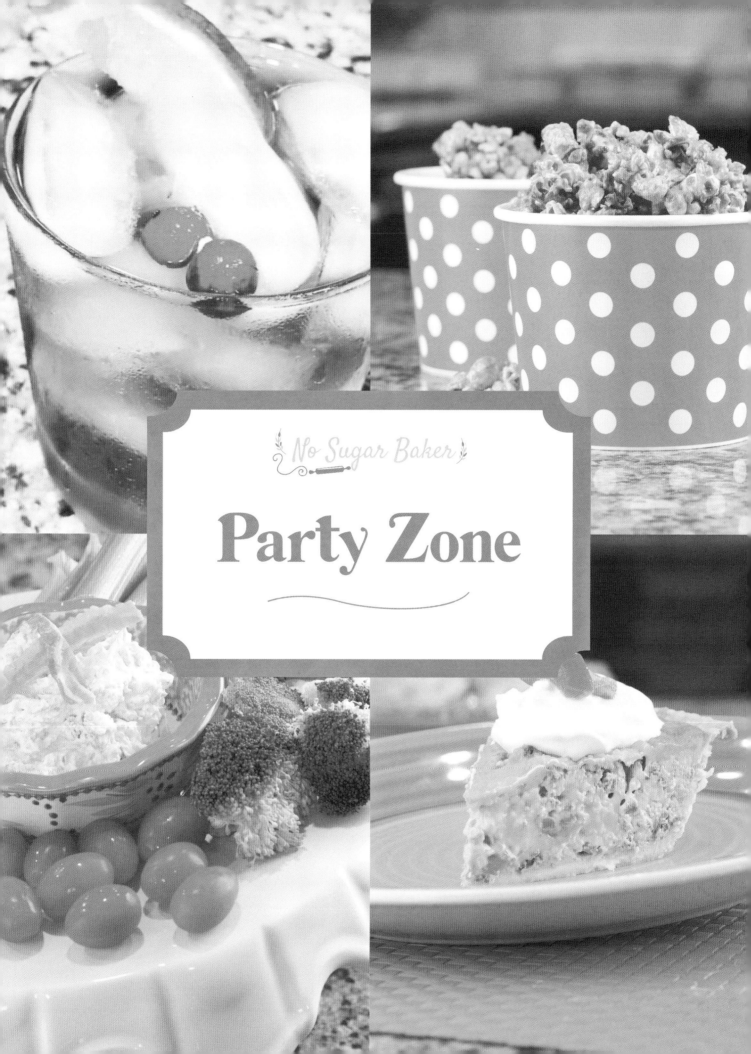

No Sugar Baker

Party Zone

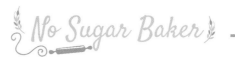
No Sugar Baker's Oh La La La The Hubs' Drinky Drink

Ingredients:

Ice Cubes
1 Oz. Lime Vodka
1 C. Sugar Free Cranberry Juice
Lime Slices
Cranberries

Easy Directions:

1. Put ice cubes in your favorite cocktail glass. Add vodka and juice. Garnish with lime slices and cranberries. Then, say oh la la la!

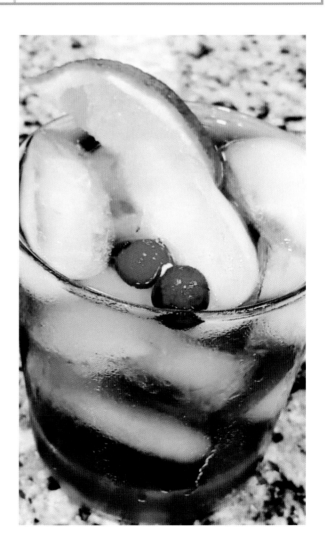

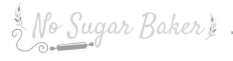
Party Zone

No Sugar Baker's
Peanut Butter Cups

Ingredients:

1 ½ C. Deli Fresh Peanut Butter

1 C. Swerve Confectioners

2 C. Lily's Dark Chocolate Chips, Melted

Easy Directions:

1. In a small bowl, combine peanut butter and Swerve. Line a mini-cupcake pan with paper liners.

2. Carefully spoon a layer of melted chocolate into each liner and spoon a spoonful of peanut butter mixture.

3. Top with remaining chocolate. Place in freezer overnight!

No Sugar Baker's Bacon Dip

Ingredients:

8 Oz. Cream Cheese
1 C. Cooked Bacon (I used bacon crumbles)
½ C. Mayonnaise

½ C. Chopped Onion
1 C. Shredded Cheese

Easy Directions:

1. In a small mixing bowl, combine all ingredients. Spread into a baking dish/pan.

2. Top with extra shredded cheese and any remaining bacon. Bake at 350 for 15 minutes.

3. Enjoy with celery, cauliflower, no sugar/low carb crackers or no sugar/low carb baked tortillas.

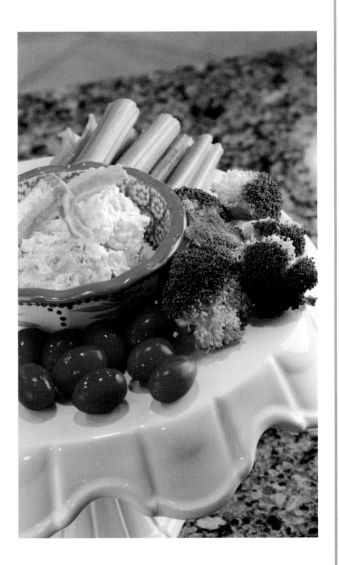

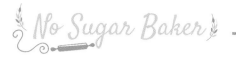

No Sugar Baker's
Buffalo Chicken Party Dip

Ingredients:

8 Oz. Cream Cheese
¾ C. Buffalo Hot Sauce
2 Cooked Chicken Breasts Diced
1 C. Shredded Cheese

Easy Directions:

1. In a small mixing bowl, combine cream cheese, hot sauce and chicken.

2. Spread into a baking dish/pan. Top with shredded cheese. Bake at 350 for 15 minutes.

3. Enjoy with celery, cauliflower, no sugar/low carb crackers or no sugar/low carb baked tortillas.

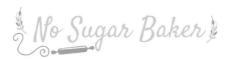

No Sugar Baker's
Blueberry Pie Ice Cream

Pie Crust Ingredients:
½ C. Almond Flour
½ C. Unsweetened Coconut
½ C. Chopped Pecans
4 T. Swerve Granular
1 t. Cinnamon
½ t. Salt
3 T. Melted Butter
1 t. Vanilla

Blueberry Sauce Ingredients:
1 ½ C. Frozen Blueberries
½ C. Water
½ C. Swerve Granular

1 T. Lemon Juice
¼ t. Xanthan Gum
4 Oz. Cream Cheese

Ice Cream Ingredients:
8 Oz. Cream Cheese
2 ½ C. Heavy Whipping Cream
1 C. Unsweetened Almond Milk
⅔ C. Swerve Granular
4 Egg Yolks
2 T. Vodka
1 t. Vanilla
¼ t. Xanthan Gum

Easy Directions:

1. Make the pie crust pieces. In a mixing bowl, whisk together all crust ingredients. It will resemble course crumbs. Spread out evenly on baking sheet and bake at 300 for 20 minutes. It will be a golden brown. Let cool and then, break into pie crust crumble pieces. Set aside.

2. In a medium saucepan, combine blueberries, water and Swerve Granular. Bring to a boil and simmer for 5 minutes. Remove from heat and stir in lemon juice and xanthan gum. Let cool and set aside.

3. Set a medium sized bowl over an ice bath and set aside. Combine cream, almond milk and Granular in saucepan over medium heat. Stir until Swerve Granular dissolves and mixture reaches 170 F on a thermometer. Whisk egg yolks in bowl. Slowly add about 1 cup of the hot cream mixture, whisking continuously to temper the yolks. Slowly whisk egg yolk mixture back into cream. Cook until 180 F on a thermometer. Pour mixture into bowl set over ice bath and allow to cool 10 minutes.

4. Then wrap tightly in plastic wrap and chill for 4 hours. Remove from refrigerator. Stir in vodka and vanilla, sprinkle with xanthan gum. Mix again. Then, follow directions of your ice cream machine and canister. Once churned, pour half into storage container and drizzle with half of the blueberry sauce and pie crusts. Repeat. Freeze for 4 hours.

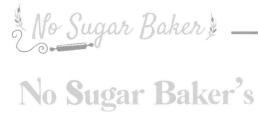

No Sugar Baker's
Caramel Popcorn

Ingredients:

2 Microwave Bags of Skinny Girl Popcorn
1 C. Butter
2 C. Swerve Brown
½ t. Salt
½ t. Vanilla

1 t. Baking Soda
½ C. Peanuts
½ C. Pecans

Easy Directions:

1. Make microwave popcorn and pour into sprayed 9 x 12 baking pan. I used an aluminum foil pan. On stovetop, in middle sized saucepan melt butter.

2. After melted, pour in Swerve and keep stirring. Bring to a boil. Reduce heat, continuing to stir for an additional 5-6 minutes.

3. Add in salt and vanilla. Remove from heat. Stir. Add in baking soda. Stir. Your caramel mixture will nearly double and became lighter in color. Pour ¼ of mixture over popcorn and stir.

4. Pour another ¼ of mixture over popcorn and stir. Bake at 300 degrees, watching the popcorn closely for browning.

5. Stirring every 7-9 minutes. Bake until the popcorn is almost dry. I bake my popcorn for 20 minutes.

6. Pour onto parchment paper, spreading out popcorn. Add in peanuts and pecans. Let dry.

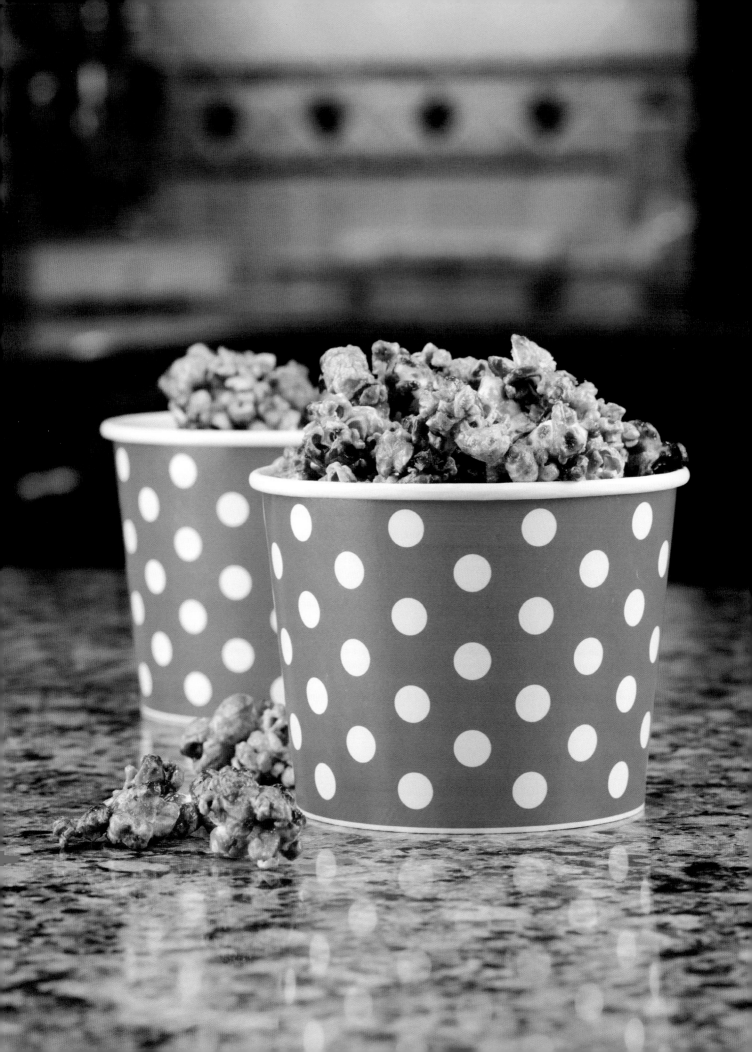

Baking Station 3:

Meet the No Sugar Baker Team

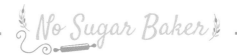

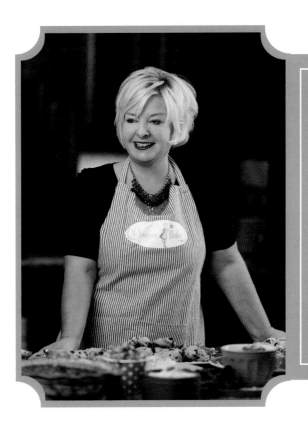

Meet the No Sugar Baker:

Jayne J. Jones Beehler
(AKA The No Sugar Baker)

Favorite Food:

Fish

Favorite Once a Year Treat:

Cheetos, Tator-tots, and I love my mom's peanut butter chocolate graham cracker or lemon bars.

Jayne, born and raised in Minnesota, grew up on chewy tator-tot-hotdish and sugary pans of bars. After law school, Jayne worked in state and federal government public policy roles. Jayne has founded a government grant firm, a nonprofit chaperone travel service for individuals with intellectual disabilities and learning differences and authored six national and world award-winning books. Jayne loves braised current events, is bubbly strong willed, and her least favorite charred word is "no." Jayne is a proud non-coffee drinking Lutheran, who drenches the church with her voice singing all hymns.

A self-taught decadent cook, baker and party thrower, Jayne's main love is entertaining and knocking everyone's aprons off with her creativity, devotion to dollar saving tips and delightful savory tastes. Though far from "a-typical," a typical weekend would find Jayne roaming enticing garage sales, trying a new gratifying recipe on her glorified taste testing team, and rooting for her friends in the National Hockey League.

Jayne got deathly ill in the fall of 2019. Her love of the kitchen, party throwing and zest for life got crumbled up in one bite. But, not out of sight. She had a sour after-taste but that bitterness won't last long or become over baked.

After six months of blood, sweat and tears, Jayne rolled up her sleeves, put back on an apron and went to work as the No Sugar Baker.

Jayne is married to Chris Beehler, (AKA The Hubs), and has a college-aged daughter Emily (AKA Em).

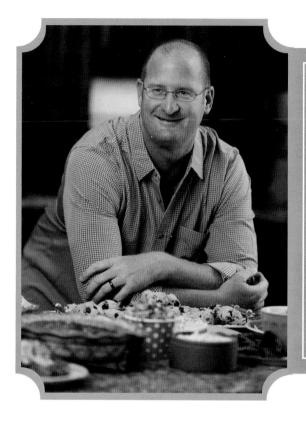

Meet the No Sugar Baker Team:

Chris Beehler
(AKA The Hubs)

The Sous Chef

Favorite Food:

Ahi Tuna or Bone-In Ribeye (Medium Rare on Both)

Favorite Once a Year Treat:
Peanut Butter Chocolate Ice Cream

Chris was born and raised in California. As a hockey goalie, he moved to the Midwest following his love of the game. Chris graduated from college with a degree in recreation management, has coached youth teams for over twenty-years and has never tasted a meal he hasn't liked.

Jayne and Chris married in 2012. He didn't know at the time; he was adventuring on a life journey with the No Sugar Baker. Chris' favorite dish is a no sugar, no flour home-made pizza. From day one of diagnosis, Chris has played a vital role in Jayne's health, ensuring her daily needed nutrition, zest for life is joyfully engaged, and giving a truthful evaluation of every new recipe.

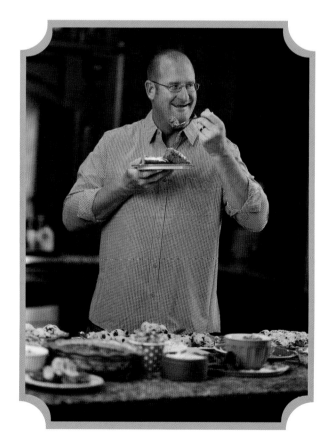

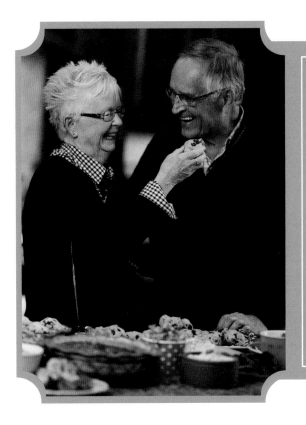

Meet the No Sugar Baker Team:

David and Margaret Jones
(AKA The Folks)

Captains of the Taste Tester Team

Favorite Food:

David: Baby Back Ribs and Any Flavor of Pie
Margaret: Porterhouse Steak Or Bowl of Buttered Noodles

Favorite Once a Year Treat:

They Share an Entire Rhubarb Meringue Pie

David and Margaret Jones have three grown children and eight grandchildren. They met as high school sweethearts and have been married for over fifty-five years. Their children have been their number one priority in life and will always remain their concern, worry and love. Jayne is their only daughter and baby of the family. The trio (The Folks plus Jayne) has been a strong unit and team from day one. They have been Jayne's sounding board on this journey and gleefully volunteer to taste test any new recipe.

They cried and thanked the Lord, the day when Jayne reintroduced herself to her kitchen. They have never missed a meal in their life and relish on sitting back watching this journey continue and unfold.

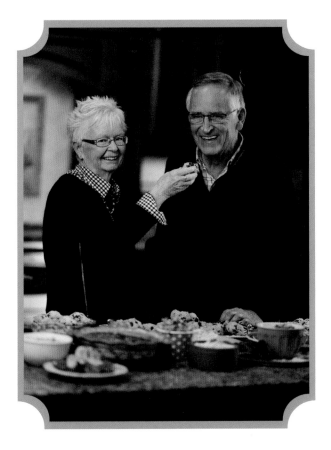

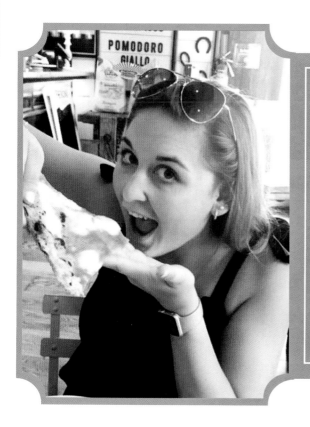

Meet the No Sugar Baker Team:

Emily Beehler
(AKA Em)

Taste Tester

Favorite Food:

Salmon and Sushi

Favorite Once a Year Treat:
Chunky Monkey Ice Cream

Emily graduated as a two-sport college athlete and is employed as a full-time police officer. Emily gets excited to try anything new, from new art projects to finding nature's coolest discoveries, Emily always has a smile.

Emily has changed her lifestyle adapting to her parents' new nutritional habits. While still a sugar junkie, Emily hasn't shied away from trying and experimenting with new sugar free recipes.

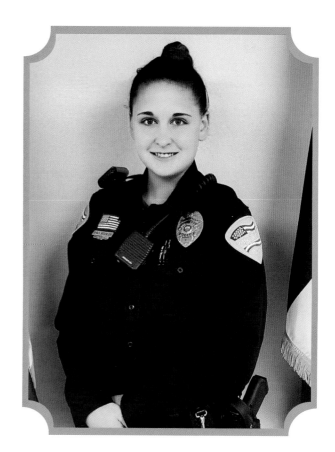

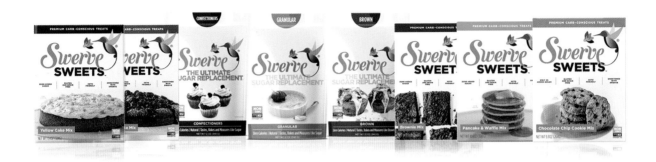

Swerve is focused on creating better-for-you baking and cooking products that are delicious and natural. We offer zero calorie sweeteners, low carb and gluten-free bake mixes, and down-to-earth education, giving everyone the tools to make their sweetest dreams come true.

Find Swerve
Lucky for you, you can find Swerve products at most major grocery stores, including Whole Foods, Walmart, and Target. Use our store locator at https://swervesweet.com/find-swerve to find Swerve near you.

Just for No Sugar Baker Fans
Email hello@swervesweetener.com for a coupon.
Please include the subject line: No Sugar Baker Coupon.